Praise for
No Manual? No Problem!

"*No Manual, No Problem* is a one-stop shop to help children and their parents thrive in our supercharged, hyperactive, faster-than-the-speed-of-light world. Spanning a range of topics from the developing brain to parenting styles to how to best read a book with your kid, Monica Reinhard-Gorney and Perk Musacchio help us manage the torrent of information on child rearing and provide a clear path to parenting that offers sound advice nurtured through years of experience."

—Kathy Hirsh-Pasek, Ph.D.
Stanley and Debra Lefkowitz Faculty Fellow, Department of Psychology, Temple University
Author of *Einstein Never Used Flash Cards* and *Becoming Brilliant*

"With an unprecedented number of children diagnosed with chronic health, learning and developmental conditions, parents in the 21st century really do need a manual. Perk and Monica have created THE manual to guide parents through the complex maze of parenting in the 21st century. By offering practical tips and strategies to overcome the root causes of our children's health and learning problems they offer hope and inspiration for every parent."

—Beth Lambert
Author of *A Compromised Generation* and *Brain Under Attack*
Executive Director, Epidemic Answers and the Documenting Hope Project

"Monica and Perk have done a wonderful job of touching on a vast number of topics that impact children, their health and their ability to learn. I am impressed that they covered topics as diverse as methylation, nutrigenomics, and the need for zinc and other nutrients to the power of positive affirmations. I think this book will be a comprehensive guide to parents on a wide range of topics to help support healthier children, both in mind as well as body!"

—Dr. Amy Yasko, Ph.D., NHD, AMD, HHP, FAAIM
Author of *AUTISM: Pathways to Recovery, Feel Good Nutrigenomics: Your Roadmap to Health,* and *Feel Good Nucleotides*

"No Manual? No Problem! takes passion, expertise, research and real-life applications and creates a comprehensive manual for parents, educators and anyone who cares about the life and development of a child. The authors have done an outstanding job considering all the factors that impact the growth of a child, making sure the 'whole child' is understood. By including data, knowledge and experience, the authors enable the reader to fully understand how the child's biology, environment and cultural norms can help the child be successful, or tear that child down. A great source for answering why our children are not thriving and what we can do?!"

—Karen L. Dickinson, Ph.D.
West Chester University Associate Professor in Counselor Education
Professional School Counselor

"Perk and Monica have written a tremendously valuable book for any parent and educator. These two uniquely experienced authors have taken on and accomplished a monumental task; illuminating and introducing a wide variety of present concerns, risks and opportunities when raising children in today's unique world. Whether they are examining risks and rewards of screen time, the need for play, specific learning struggles or the uniqueness of the adolescent brain, both authors understand the need for looking at current research and keeping focused on emotional and family health in easy to understand ways. Brava for combining heart with mind, no easy task."

—Sanford Shapiro, M.Ed.
Learning Specialist and Educational Consultant

"Parents are a child's first and most important teachers. But unlike professional educators, parents, as a rule, receive little training. Most of us rely on what our parents did for us and what our friends with children our children's ages think and do. Most of the time, for most of us, things seem to work out. But some of us most of the time and all of us some of the time, are not sure what to do or to whom to turn when we need advice. In No Manual? No Problem! two experienced educator/parents -- Monica Reinhard-Gorney and Perk Musacchio—help bridge the gap between parent and educator with some strategies for helping our children thrive in today's challenging world. They identify a number of "culprits" which may be inhibiting our children's success and present a number of options we may consider for arresting those culprits.

No Manual? No Problem! is written in straightforward language without reliance on the esoteric language of educators. It's written by parents for parents in language parents will find "no problem." The book offers no guarantees. But it does offer some hope in the form of new approaches to old problems and some resources for those who may need them. In reading this book I was encouraged to think about old things in new ways and to consider things I'd never considered before. Now that's a book worth reading."

—Joseph E. Haviland
Professor at Temple University

"*No Manual? No Problem!* is a 'must read' manual which identifies current trends and profiles multiple barriers to optimizing child development and learning, and is for anyone who has or works with children e.g. parents, teachers, school admin, clinicians, counsellors, psychologists and physicians."

—Cris Rowan, BScOT, BScBi, SIPT
CEO Sunshine Coast Occupational Therapy Inc. and Zone'in Programs Inc.
Author of *Virtual Child: The terrifying truth about what technology is doing to children*

"I write this not just as a clinical neuroscientist and a university professor but most importantly as the parent of a toddler. The western society and lifestyle is plagued with technological riches. We live in a time where playtime is being prescribed to children and adolescents. Where we (and our children) are consumed by technology and screen time. Where there is so much information overload the brain doesn't have time to decompress, relax, untether...detox. So, the audience of this book should not just be those seeking answers and information on their academically or otherwise underperforming child, but any parent, educator, and counselor. This information is for all. Written by two very distinguished educators with significant experience. The book makes a great informational read. A manual if I may...no manual, no problem! Here it is. Well rounded information on the what, when, where, and hows. Kudos to the authors on this book and must read for any parent (not) looking for answers."

—Harsimran S Baweja P.T. Ph.D.
Associate Professor, Physical Therapy, Applied Movement Sciences, and Substance Abuse Director, Neuromechanics and Neuroplasticity LaboratorySchool of Exercise and Nutritional SciencesCollege of Health and Human Services at San Diego State University

No Manual?
No Problem!

No Manual?
No Problem!

Strategies and Interventions to
Help Your Child Thrive in Today's World

Monica Reinhard-Gorney, MS.ED.

Perk Musacchio, M.ED.

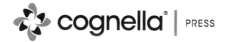 cognella® | PRESS

First published in the United States of America in 2019 by Cognella, Inc.

Cover image copyright© 2016 iStockphoto LP/Kudryashka.
Cover design by Emely Villavicencio

Printed in the United States of America

ISBN: 978-1-5165-3418-0 (pbk)

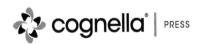 PRESS

www.cognella.com   800-200-3908

Contents

SECTION III: THE OPTIONS

Monica

To Ava—my greatest teacher. To Dr. Bill Gagliardi and Sue Fisher Mustalish, who got the ball rolling in the right direction. To Dr. Daphne Goldberg, Michlyn Gazaway, and Dr. Amy Yasko—my heroes, my angels—your unwavering bravery and natural instincts to help others changed our path forever. To my sister Sharon—you gave me strength when I needed it most. To Rob, Ava, and Cora—you make every day a gift. To Barb Messaros, Heather Evans, and Jenny Tyler —my sounding boards. To my mom and dad, Krystal, and the Gorneys who helped along the way. To the faculty of Bryn Mawr College who instill the courage to ask the "how" and "why" questions. To Cara Frank, Dr. Seth Koss, Dr. Peter Prociuk, Dr. Janet McGaurn, Dr. Chaya Herzberg, Tricia Holowsko, Chris Madden, Holly and Todd Grimm, Dr. Chris Hannafin, Dr. Elizabeth Webb, Maude LeRoux, Angela Gaudiuso Johnson, and the staff at ATA, you each possess a natural talent for what you do—you educate, you empower, and you offer hope and a path! To past and present students and parents—you all share the journey so openly and honestly, it is always an honor to collaborate with you!

Perk

To my family—each of whom has taught me different lessons that have made me a better teacher. I learned to appreciate the "outside the box" thinkers, those with a quirky sense of humor, and that moving to learn is critical for some. I learned to get to the root of a problem and not just treat the symptoms. I learned and continue to learn that life is all about compromise, flexibility, and forgiveness. To Clif Beaver—one of the best principals and human beings ever! I am forever grateful for your belief in me, your willingness to allow me to seek out new information and programs, and your blessings to take what I learned to help our students reach their true potential. To my colleagues—"It's a beautiful thing when a career and a passion come together." That quote perfectly describes my 40+ years in education. I am truly blessed to have taught with you and consider you to be my dear friends and true supporters. To my students—you made it all worthwhile. Your smiles, your hugs, your "aha" moments, and even the tears and struggles. For it is those struggles and frustrations that taught me patience and to never say "never" until I had answers and could help you succeed.

From Monica and Perk

To all our readers—may you and your children have healthy, successful, and joyous lives. To Kassie Graves for believing in our work. To Natalie Lakosil and Alisa Muñoz—for the countless hours, the guidance, and for helping make this book a reality.

Introduction

> "The human race should just slow down
> and think about what it is doing."
>
> —Michael Palin

Something is happening to children. What is happening has been slow and subtle, so much so that you may not have noticed unless you had been working with children every day in the classroom for several decades, or unless you were a high school counselor who also happens to be a parent of a child who had a dramatic health scare and recovery. Our experiences have allowed us to observe the ways that children and teens have changed, and we want to share what we have witnessed because we believe what we have seen has an impact on all children and families.

Whether you are reading this book because you are a parent to be, the parent of young children yet to attend school, the parent of a child with struggles, or any combination in between, our hope is that we share the common goal of wanting to see all children reach their potential, and that you'd like to see our world be a safer and more supportive place for children. We share some concerning information in this book about the hurdles that face children and families today; however, we also share important tools that all parents can utilize to maximize their child's development and some revolutionary interventions for children who need more help. This book is a manual for parents - educator and mother designed.

During the last 20 years, the school setting has changed dramatically. At the elementary level, the prevalence of developmental and learning challenges has been noticeably rising, with more and more children struggling with language acquisition, vocabulary, reading, comprehension, fine and gross motor skills, and general problem-solving. Furthermore, children are increasingly being treated for social, emotional, physical, and mental health issues.

These issues, when unaddressed, become all the more challenging at the secondary level when the stakes are higher and attached to outcomes such as college and career placement. It seems that an increased number of teens are struggling to meet the demands made of them in high school and college, even those enrolled in Advanced Placement (AP) courses. We have noticed a specific decline in critical-thinking skills and the ability to be self-reflective, both of which must be demonstrated to be successful in the college essay and interview process. We have also experienced a growing number of teens being treated for emotional problems such as cutting and self-medicating. For teens who have been prescribed medication for diagnoses such as attention deficit disorder (ADD), depression, or anxiety, the potential negative side effects, such as severe fluctuations in weight or sleep disturbances, create additional hurdles to physical and emotional well-being and/or academic success.

To accommodate the growing number of students with challenges or limitations, many schools are hiring more special education staff, school counselors, and nurses. Districts have even begun employing school social workers, behavior specialists, and therapists (i.e., occupational therapists, physical therapists, and speech and language therapists). Several decades ago, many of these positions didn't exist, were shared between buildings, or the services were contracted out. As the number of students who require these services increases, it becomes necessary, and sometimes financially prudent, for schools to staff from within and provide more ongoing support.

While we frequently discussed these complex and unsettling changes with our colleagues, we also independently experienced certain events in our personal and professional lives that left us with the drive to find solutions to all these problems.

Monica

My early work with teens included serving as a counselor in a day treatment program for at-risk youth, an admissions counselor in a boarding school, and a guidance counselor in a top-ranked public high school. I enjoy helping teens find strength and courage in their own voice, while also helping them determine where the future might take them. However, with an overwhelming caseload, limitations on how I could help students in a public school setting, and the desire to start a family of my own, I decided that transitioning into private practice would be a good career move.

In the early summer of 2005, my husband and I were thrilled to learn that we were expecting our first child. I already ate well and exercised regularly before I was pregnant, and all my visits to the doctor and routine tests indicated everything with the pregnancy and baby was fine. So, of course we were totally unprepared for the shock and challenges we experienced when our daughter became very ill shortly after birth.

Her symptoms were many; she became increasingly covered in eczema from head to toe and had rashes so itchy that she scratched until she bled. She had horrible acid reflux and was prescribed two acid reflux medications to help her tolerate the medical formula that she was living on, yet she was barely in the 10th percentile for weight. Our attempts to introduce solid food were met with one food allergy diagnosis after the next. She hardly slept, and on many days she cried half the day or more. Her muscle tone was poor, and over time she became limp and even despondent. The best explanation that the specialists at one of the top children's hospitals offered us was, "your daughter was just born this way."

My husband and I asked ourselves constantly how our daughter could be so sick. Neither of us had any health issues, nor did anyone in our immediate families, and three out of my four grandparents lived into their 90s! Everything about these major medical interventions felt intuitively wrong, and our daughter was only getting worse, not better. Because she was so ill, she had developed a myriad of other issues since she was too weak to physically engage in all the typical activities babies, toddlers, and young children do that are critical for development. For example, her stomach muscles were so weak that she could not sit up independently until she was a year old. When we went to the park, her hands and feet, and sometimes her airway, swelled in reaction to the mold that is found in most mulches. Because we avoided parks, she never learned to climb on playground equipment like other children, and this impacted the development of her gross motor skills. Her fingers and hands would swell up when she touched playdough or crayons, which we later learned was a reaction to the gluten and dyes found in those products. With a lack of things to manipulate, her fine motor skills also lagged behind. We were ever-challenged and incredibly disheartened by the struggles that our daughter faced and the fact that we could not seem to find solutions, until we met an integrative medical doctor.

The integrative medical doctor took a much deeper look at our daughter's situation and offered explanations for what she determined to be the underlying causes of our daughter's illness, and better yet, she was able to direct us to other health practitioners and treatments that could help her. It was only when we started implementing the recommended treatment plans of these doctors and practitioners that we started to see great improvements in our daughter's health.

The physical health aspect of her regimen was driven by a genetically based protocol aimed at addressing underlying gut and immune weaknesses. This involved preparing a daily concoction of specific vitamins, minerals, and supplements and then tracking her progress through various blood, urine, and stool tests. She was on this regimen for 3 years, and now, 10 years later, she only takes a fraction of those supplements daily to maintain her health. This part of the program was occasionally enhanced by a visit to our homeopathic doctor who prescribed various remedies to help with challenges that arose throughout her treatment. She also had weekly acupuncture sessions on and off for about a year, the goal of which was to calm her overreacting immune system. Once her gut and immune system were in better balance, over a two-year period we employed some of the techniques shared in chapter 10 to strengthen her fine and gross motor and executive function skills, which had been weakened or poorly established due to her physical health challenges.

I don't share my daughter's story because I think that her overall experience is common, but because I was blown away that there were solutions to everyday problems that even I, as a highly trained educator, had never heard of. Through her experience, we learned that there are known root causes for many of the health, developmental, and learning challenges that children are diagnosed with and not limited to the ones our daughter faced. Viable treatments are available that can greatly improve, if not reverse, some of these conditions. Remember that poor muscle tone I mentioned my daughter had? Well, it turns out that was a global situation. I had no idea how many muscles were involved in two eyes being able to look at information in a book and read. But once it was identified in first grade that she had poor and uncoordinated eye muscles, she did a three-month course of vision therapy aimed at building the strength of those muscles and training them to work together. During that time, she learned to read. That was without any special reading instruction, and she is now an advanced reader. I wondered how many children struggling to read had a visual weakness and not a reading problem, and why it wasn't standard protocol to suggest a developmental pediatric eye exam (which is different than a regular vision exam) before suggesting reading remediation. Remember the acid reflux and the dozens of food allergies? By strengthening her gut and immune system, the acid reflux is now totally gone, and only a couple of food allergies remain. Before seeing this doctor, we felt like we had been handed a life sentence, then we discovered, at least in our case, that it didn't need to be that way.

During the time that I sat in the waiting rooms of the clinics we frequented, I came to learn about children diagnosed with dyslexia who were told they would never read without assistance, who learned to read independently. I saw heavily medicated kids with debilitating ADHD, lose their ADHD diagnoses and cease medication following biomedical treatment or neurofeedback. I saw children with life-threatening hospitalizations for asthma, no longer even need an inhaler following dietary changes. Our daughter is now thriving physically and emotionally and is earning top grades in above-grade-level courses without special education. She is enrolled in four dance classes a week and has a full and well-rounded life. Those who had not witnessed her early years would never believe she had so many struggles.

It was around the time that my daughter was healing that I decided to reach out to someone whom I had known many years before. Back in 2000, Perk and I both worked in the same public school district. We initially encountered one another because I was Perk's son's guidance counselor, but over time we attended certain district trainings together and became friends. Once I left the district, our paths only crossed on occasion. I knew Perk was still in the trenches with elementary children, and I was curious to know if she was aware of all the interventions and therapies that I had learned about.

Perk shared what she and her colleagues had been observing. There was an increasing number of children who required intensive help and yet seemed to be resistant to the tried-and-true strategies that had worked in the past and an increasing complexity of their diagnoses and struggles. She also shared that she had a great revelation regarding children's development, and what she learned was so profound that she began shifting gears in her approach to working with children.

Perk

Upon reflecting on the troubling things I was seeing in the schools where I had taught for the past 30 years, I began to question myself. Had I become less patient with students? Was I falling short and not providing appropriate instruction for my students? Why weren't the students coming to school with the same level of skills that they had years before? There was a disconnect that I couldn't explain. As I talked to other educators, both new and veteran, I discovered that everyone was observing the same things, and they were just as concerned. My philosophy has always been that there are alternate routes around any roadblock that prevents students from being successful. With an open mind, I continually researched and regularly collaborated with other professionals to find creative solutions for our struggling students.

In 2005, I had the opportunity to attend an international conference in Boston where I met world-renowned physicians, neuroscientists, educators, and psychiatrists who presented on many current topics about brain development, such as the importance of play, the effects of technology on the developing brain, the stress that overscheduling can create, and parenting styles that can really make a difference. The presentations were enlightening but startling at the same time. The research was showing that real changes were occurring in the brains of children. The pieces of the puzzle began to slowly come together for me; I wasn't necessarily doing anything wrong, but rather something was different with students.

I returned from that conference more passionate than ever because now I knew why we were seeing the same trends among students at our school as doctors, educators, psychologists, and therapists were seeing nationwide. I felt that we, as educators, had to figure out a way to address as many of the issues we could in the classroom, knowing there is much that was beyond our control. My colleagues and I implemented some of the strategies presented in this book that are appropriate for the classroom environment, and for a few years we saw some improvements. However, if steps to improve overall development, health, and well-being were not continued in the home, we soon realized that our efforts in isolation were no better than a Band-Aid.

When Monica and I reconnected, we knew that we needed to come up with a way to share our knowledge and experience with parents and educators everywhere, because we feel strongly that a more global and holistic approach to parenting and education will remedy many of the physical, learning, and emotional challenges children face today. This is why we wrote this book.

Our Hope

We understand that parents are bombarded with a lot of information, and when compartmentalized by topic it may seem like these problems exist in isolation and are only relevant to some. However, our book addresses the cumulative problem, because when you look at all of the things in our world that are having an impact on children, their development, and their success in the classroom and beyond, the problem becomes significant, and in some cases, we'd even say staggering.

Being a parent or an educator has never been easy, but it is even more challenging in today's world, because the reality is that our world, our classrooms, and children have changed. Consider, for example, how different the life of a 6-month-old, a 5-year-old, or a teenager is now than it was just a couple decades ago. Infants and toddlers can be seen holding and manipulating devices such as iPads, sometimes for hours at a time. Concern about the cumulative impact of radiation from those devices is now making headlines.

As a result of the increasing number of school shootings and violence, concern about the physical safety of our children has led to significant changes in schools. For example, when attempting to enter most schools, visitors will almost always be met by a locked door and maybe even a high-tech security system. After being buzzed in, they will be asked to supply their identification, and if the visitors are there to volunteer, they will have to provide clearances, which are documents that show they do not have a criminal background. Monthly drills have always been held for weather alerts, but now intruder and lockdown drills are also practiced, even by children in preschool and elementary school.

Mental health issues are on the rise. In the last few years, more than a few teenagers have live-streamed their suicides on social media, in most instances the footage has been seen by thousands of teens before being taken down. Dozens of teens nationwide have posted their suicide notes on social media before taking their lives, and children are often spreading the word of their deaths via text before parents and school administrators even know the news or can take any sort of action to buffer children from the trauma of these losses.

Our food supply has become very controversial, and food allergies are on the rise. In 2016, Congress passed the Dark Act, which allows food manufacturers to choose whether they want to share with you that the food you and your children are eating has been genetically modified. Many infant and toddler foods now contain genetically modified ingredients, except you don't necessarily know it. Most of the countries in the European Union have banned genetically modified foods from their food supply due to what they feel is a lack of evidence of their safety. Also, recent research has revealed the hazards of a low- or nonfat food diet, which many children are consuming.

Other unsettling facts that reflect the way our children's experience in society have changed include: children are becoming more sedentary and childhood obesity is on the rise; there is now a diagnosis for device or gaming addiction; and in 2014 the Centers for

Disease Control and Prevention (CDC) reported that over 10,000 toddlers, ages 2 to 3 years, are on stimulant medications for ADHD alone.[1]

Adding to this troublesome landscape is the prominence of social media and the opportunity to always be plugged in due to ever-evolving technology, which also provides an arena outside of school for things like cyberbullying. Former Facebook president, Sean Parker, said that Facebook "literally changes your relationship with society, with each other." Parker continued to say that the social media giant creates "a social-validation feedback loop" that exploits a core vulnerability in the human psyche. "God only knows what it's doing to our children's brains."[2] Chamath Palihapitiya, the former head of Facebook's user growth division said, "The short-term, dopamine-driven feedback loops that we have created are destroying how society works."[3]

The reality is that all of these issues have an impact on children and their ability to function. While many pediatricians share concern over some of the topics in this book, the current mainstream model of healthcare in this country barely affords a pediatrician time to address important physical health topics during a wellness check-up. And, unfortunately, the government's primary solution to the declining performance of children has been to change the nature of educational curriculum and instruction, funding programs like the Common Core, No Child Left Behind, and its recent replacement, the Every Child Succeeds Act. More and longer school days, ramped up grade-level expectations, standards that are often developmentally inappropriate, high-stakes testing, and monster loads of homework are creating an unprecedented level of student and familial stress.

The fact is that this approach is a narrow and one-dimensional analysis of a multidimensional problem. This approach does not take into account other factors, or "culprits," as we refer to them in this book, that are having an impact on children's overall health and well-being, which ultimately impacts academic performance. We've identified five culprits that interfere with a child's optimal developmental trajectory and discuss them in greater detail in chapters 4, 5, 6, and 7. They are:

- Inadequate nutrition

- Environmental toxins

- Lack of unstructured and creative play

- Overuse of screens and technology

- Overscheduled, busy lifestyles

Scientific studies are now confirming what we suspected about these culprits. For example, we are now learning that some of the information we once thought to be healthy is actually not, such as depriving the body of certain fats, which is encouraged by the plethora of low- or nonfat food products on the shelves; this type of diet alters hormone production and overall health. A lack of active and imaginative play is impacting brain and body development. While many news headlines would lead you to believe that technology is the best thing in the world for our children and their learning, research shows that too much time on screens is actually changing the careful balance of neurotransmitters in the brain.

While we can't change everything about our environment and culture, we must understand and remember that we can have some control over the impact of these culprits in our lives. The information in this book has the potential to invaluably change the lives of children because informed parents can make better decisions. In our early chapters, we offer a common foundation of knowledge about the brain and child development so that all parents can have a better understanding of how their children should be developing. Then, with a more solid understanding of the brain, parents can make better sense of the information on the culprits that we feel have the potential to derail ideal social, emotional and cognitive development. We provide research on different parenting styles so that parents can learn the often times predictable relationship between parental and child behavior. Later we share essential building blocks for social, emotional and academic success, and over 100 strategies to foster that development.

We also offer effective strategies that you can implement in your home that can ease the challenges you may be facing with your child's learning and/or behavior. Finally, we introduce you to more involved interventions and therapies that can be implemented with the help of professionals to dramatically improve the symptoms associated with many learning disabilities or emotional and behavioral diagnoses. Much of the information we share is grounded in the scientific principle of neuroplasticity, which means that while the brain may have been wired a certain way at birth, it undergoes many changes throughout the course of a person's development and is even capable of healing and changing through participation in certain interventions and treatments.

Now, more than ever, parents need trusted resources, and children need us to step up and make positive change happen. Our hope is that you come away from this book feeling empowered, because with the proper knowledge, everyone can be a part of the solution—this book is just the beginning.

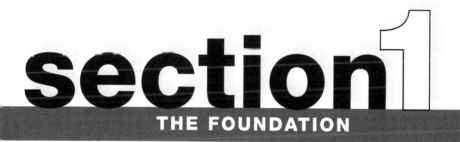

section1

THE FOUNDATION

Chapter one

Alarming Statistics

"Let's raise children who won't have to recover from their childhoods."

—Pam Leo

The data shared in this chapter shows that the rate of learning and physical and mental health based diagnoses is, in fact, increasing. Not only is this distressing for the children and parents who are affected, but the rising rate of these issues strains every classroom and the entire school system.

As we shared in our introduction, we have seen significant changes in our schools and student performance. According to *U.S. News & World Report* and *Newsweek*, our own local Pennsylvania schools are ranked as some of the most excellent schools in the country. However, despite that ranking, amazing programming, systematic and multisensory instruction, excellent support services, and high standards and expectations for all students, the rate of children receiving special education services has never been higher.

Soon we will share some statistics on the rising rates of many diagnoses impacting children, but first we wanted to address a popular argument made that some things only seem worse because we are simply more knowledgeable, more aware, or because better diagnostic tools are now available. While this may be the case in some instances, we don't believe that to be so with most issues that we see impacting children today. For example, the incidence of anaphylactic food allergies is higher than ever before. Thirty years ago it was rare for there to be multiple EpiPens® in a nurse's office, and bags of EpiPens® didn't go on field trips with kids. It is highly unlikely that school personnel, or doctors for that matter, simply overlooked or could not identify children going into anaphylactic shock—there simply just weren't as many children affected by these severe allergies.

Back in the early 1990s, in one particular school district, there was an increase in the rate of students who were being identified for special education in the category of "specific reading disability." The administration and the teachers knew, per educational statistics, that no more than 4 percent of the student population should require special education. If more than 4 percent of the student population required special education, then the school should look at the general education programs, because something must be faulty in curriculum or instruction. It was decided that a different reading program should be taught to all primary students, and following the implementation of the new reading program the number of students being diagnosed with that specific reading disability began to decrease. That is what happens when you address the root cause of a problem. When rising rates of disability are due to poor programming or instruction, you fix the source of the problem, and you see improvement. We wish we could say that the percentage of students receiving special education has remained lower, but it hasn't. For example, in our state of Pennsylvania the rate has quadrupled, and is now at 15.9 percent.

The big question becomes, why? We feel that despite excellent educational programming more and more children are having learning, emotional, and neurological challenges that don't fit into any particular category, and their challenges are becoming more complex. Ask any daycare worker, educator (preschool to college), nurse, therapist, or anyone who has worked with children for more than 20 years; something is different. The needs are greater and not so clear-cut. Some of the needs are so great that school districts and/or local agencies assign personal care assistants or behavior specialists to children who need continuous adult support throughout the school day. In our home state of Pennsylvania alone, this greater need is reflected in the education budget for the 2017–2018 school year. The general education budget rose by 1.7 percent over the previous year, yet the special education budget increased by 2.3 percent over the previous year.[1] Considering that the number of students receiving special education is drastically less than the number of students in the general education population, as in 16 percent to 84 percent, it is eye-opening that the budget costs for special education are escalating at a rate greater than that for the general education population.

Undoubtedly, there is a relationship between children's physical, mental, and neurological health and their performance at school. We wanted to know if our more personal and local observation that children seemed to be struggling with more issues was backed by national trends and data. The data we uncovered substantiates that children across the country are experiencing greater physical, mental, and cognitive challenges.

Physical Health

Allergies

Food allergies are at an all-time high. They increased over 400 percent from 1997 to 2007, and fatal allergies are more common than ever before.[2]

Asthma

From 1980 to 2000, the number of doctor visits for asthma nearly tripled, from 6 million annually to 17.3 million. Asthma-related deaths have increased by 56 percent (2007), and now more than 9 million American kids younger than age 18 have asthma. In 2007, asthma medical care costs were $11.5 billion annually.[3] Ten years later, in 2017, the group Documenting Hope reports that asthma costs the United States $56 billion a year.[4]

Cancer

According to the National Cancer Institute, cancer is the leading cause of death by disease past infancy. Over 10,000 new cases are diagnosed each year, and there has been a 0.06 percent increase in the rate of cancer each year for the last 35 years.[5] One in every 330 children will be diagnosed with cancer.[6]

Diabetes

Type 1 diabetes is the kind of diabetes that most doctors and researchers say children are born with and was once considered rare. The rate of type 1 diabetes has been increasing by 30 percent per decade.[7]

Type 2 diabetes accounts for the majority of diagnosed cases and is usually associated with older age, obesity, family history, physical inactivity, and race or ethnicity. It can be prevented and does respond to treatment. Until recently, type 2 diabetes was rare in people younger than 30 years. In 1990, the rate of type 2 diabetes began to surge from the 4 percent where it had held steady for decades. The leading cause of type 2 diabetes in children is obesity.[8] Researchers from the SEARCH for Diabetes in Youth study shared that the rate of Type II diabetes in 10–19 years olds rose 21 percent from 2001 to 2009.[9]

Obesity

When comparing the rate of obesity among children since 1988, we see that it is increasing at an alarming rate:

Age Range (years)	1988	2012
2 to 5 years	7.2%	10.2%
6 to 11 years	11.3%	17.9%
12 to 19 years	10%	19%

In fact, according to Beth Lambert and Victoria Kobliner, authors of *A Compromised Generation*, over one-third of American children are classified as either obese or overweight, a tripling in prevalence since the 1970s.[10]

Mental and Emotional Health

Anxiety, Depression, and Suicide

Many people experience some low-level anxiety from time to time, and this is normal. However, it crosses a line when it starts to have a significant impact on one's daily life; this is when it may become a diagnosable condition. According to statistics from the National Institute of Mental Health, the prevalence of anxiety disorders among those aged 13 to 18 years is 25.1 percent. This means that one in four teenagers has a diagnosable anxiety condition.[11]

Being exposed to a chronic source of anxiety causes some children to experience emotional trauma and may lead to a greater risk of poor physical and mental health, negative social consequences in life, and a shortened life span. In her article, "Childhood Trauma Leads to Lifelong Chronic Illness—So Why Isn't the Medical Community Helping Patients?" science reporter Donna Jackson Nakazawa revealed that two-thirds of Americans report having adverse childhood experiences (ACEs). These experiences range from extreme cases of abuse (physical and emotional), to having a parent who suffered from depression or alcoholism, divorce, or death of a loved one. Experiencing trauma makes one twice as likely to receive a costly medical diagnosis in adulthood. According to the CDC, the cost of treating patients with early childhood trauma is $124 billion annually.[12] A collaborative effort between the CDC and Kaiser Permanente revealed that in a study of 125,000 patients, those who had a doctor who acknowledged and helped them address their childhood trauma experienced a 35 percent reduction in doctor visits.[13] This is why more professionals are utilizing an ACE survey with their clients, as this questionnaire can identify those who may be at greater risk, and therefore offer early intervention and prevention.[14] Not all adverse life events can be avoided, but seeking and receiving the appropriate help following these events can greatly reduce their impact later on.[15]

Rates of depression and anxiety among young people in America have been steadily increasing for the past 50 to 70 years. James Prescott, researcher at the National Institute of Health (Child Health and Human Development), reported that 1.5 million prescriptions for antidepressants are issued annually for children under the age of 18. Suicide is the third leading cause of death for those between the ages of 15 and 24 and the fifth leading cause of death for those aged 5 to 14.[16] In 2010, counseling centers at 93 universities nationwide reported a 30 percent increase in caseloads of students with mood and anxiety disorders and suicidal ideation.[17]

In an article written for *The Conversation* in the fall of 2017, Dr. Jean Twenge summarizes the findings of a published research study that she and her colleagues conducted.[18] She says,

> Around 2012, something started going wrong in the lives of teens. In just the five years between 2010 and 2015, the number of U.S. teens who felt useless and joyless, classic symptoms of depression, surged 33 percent in large national surveys. And in fact, this large youth survey revealed that teens, who spent more time on social media and electronic devices such as smartphones, were more likely to report mental health issues.[19] Teen suicide attempts increased 23 percent. Even more troubling, the number of 13- to 18-year-olds who committed suicide jumped 31 percent.[20]

Dr. Twenge and her colleagues, using a variety of respectable methodologies, were able to rule out homework load and academic pressure as cause for increase in suicide rates. Interestingly, they found a strong correlation between the increase in female suicide rates and the use of social media.[21]

Attention Deficit Hyperactivity Disorder (ADHD)

ADHD has increased by at least 400 percent over the past 20 years. Now, more than 3.5 million children are living with the diagnosis. American children consume 90 percent of the world's Ritalin, the most popular ADHD medication. In 1997, 6.5 percent of children aged 5 to 17 were reported to have ADHD. In 2013, this rate increased to 10.1 percent.[22]

Autism

According to statistics provided by the CDC, autism has increased from approximately 1 in every 5,000 births in 1975 to 1 in 88 in 2012. Data from the National Center for Educational Statistics shows that in 1977 there were no autistic students receiving services in our schools, but in the 2013–2014 school year, 538,000 students were receiving services for autism. Given that one could argue that autism was not well known or diagnosed in 1977, we looked at the year 2000, when it was well known and diagnosed, and there were 93,000 students receiving services. Thirteen years later, there was a reported increase of 445,000 students receiving services for autism![23]

Prescription Medication Use

One of the factors that has impacted children's performance in the classroom is the increasing amount of physical and mental health problems that children face, but with that also comes the side effects of over-the-counter and prescription medications used to treat those conditions. According to data released by the CDC, in 1960 the annual expenditure on prescription medications was $2.7 billion. In 2013, that figure was $271 billion. In a little over 50 years, the amount of medication required by Americans has increased 9,937 percent. These numbers reflect the total population, but the following data are specific to children.[24]

CDC data from 2012 indicated that 7.5 percent of the population aged 6 to 17 years were on prescription medication for emotional or behavioral problems.[25] Data in *Pediatrics*, the official journal of the American Academy of Pediatrics, reveals that in 2010 more than 1.3 million prescriptions were written for adolescents for the antidepressant Sertraline and another 1.3 million prescriptions for the antidepressant Prozac.[26] The use of atypical antidepressants (antidepressants that don't fit into the category of antidepressants but act on neurotransmitters to affect symptoms of depression) rose 42 percent from 1997 to 2000.[27]

In 2002, doctors wrote 1.2 million prescriptions of antipsychotic medications for children.[28] In the three-year period from 1997 to 2000 the use of antipsychotic medication increased 138 percent.[29] A recent release of data by the CDC states that 10,000 toddlers—children aged 4 and under—are on amphetamine-based ADHD medications,[30] and 3.5 million prescriptions for ADHD medication were written for high school–aged children in 2013.[31]

Dr. Mark Hyman, medical director of the Cleveland Clinic's Center for Functional Medicine, acknowledged that, "the untested and potentially unsafe combinations of psychotropic drug cocktails has increased 500 percent in children."[32] The increase in children being treated with drugs is disheartening to say the least, but it is especially concerning to learn that a number of those drugs are not significantly or appropriately tested for safety in the ways that they are being prescribed. Rather than continue to observe these rates increase, we need to find a way to prevent this from happening in the first place.

Learning and Developmental Milestones

According to the National Center for Education Statistics, the rate of specific learning disabilities more than doubled from 1977 (1.8 percent) to 2012 (4.6 percent).[33] In their book *Learning Disabilities*, authors Roger Pierangelo and George Giuliani share that in the 24th Annual Report to Congress in 2002, the U.S. Department of Education, Office for Special Education, reported that 5 percent of the population, or 2.9 million school-aged children, had a learning disability.[34] This statistic only reflects those enrolled in public school. As there are a substantial number of private schools that solely enroll learning disabled children, many regularly estimate the number of learning disabled children to be higher. Kenneth Bock, Cameron Stauth, and Korri Fink, in their groundbreaking book, *Healing the New Childhood Epidemics*, suggest that the rate of learning disabilities within the total population (including children in private schools) is closer to 20 percent.[35]

Accommodations on Standardized Tests

The SAT uses different criteria to determine whether a student is eligible for accommodations than the ACT. But these testing companies have two things in common: (1) they require that you have a diagnosis to get accommodations, such as a specific learning disability or ADHD, and (2) the rate of students needing accommodations for each test has increased.[36]

In the 2007–2008 school year, approximately 49,767 students received accommodations on the ACT. During the 2010–2011 school year, 78,441 students received accommodations. Over the course of three school years, 28,673 more students needed accommodations.

In the 2005–2006 school year, the SAT received 70,000 requests for accommodations. In the 2010–2011 school year, they received

80,000. In other words, 10,000 more requests in a matter of five years' time.[37]

The above numbers don't include the number of students who applied for accommodations but were denied. In guidance counseling offices all across America, counselors prepare applications for extra time for their students who are receiving support and services at school, and yet some of those students are denied. If you look at the numbers above, about 7 percent of the test-takers are receiving accommodations. Therefore, 7 percent of the student population applying to college who need these tests require accommodations, and a great many more are denied. Also, many learning disabled children do not even take these tests, so it seems fair to believe that the rate of learning disabilities in the population is greater than 7 percent.

Developmental Delays

Developmental delay is a broad group of disabilities that affect major life activities such as language, mobility, learning, and self-care. The National Center for Educational Statistics reports that in 1977 there were no students receiving services for developmental delays, but in the 2013–2014 school year there were 410,000 students receiving services for delays. Again, one could argue that in 1977 developmental delay was not being diagnosed as thoroughly as it is today, so we compared the data from the years 2000 and 2013, and found that some 213,000 students were receiving services for delay in 2000,[38] and in 2013 the number of students receiving services for delay nearly doubled! According to data from the CDC, the rate of developmental disabilities increased 17 percent from 1997 to 2008.[39]

"Other Health Impairments"

In 1977, 141,000 students received services under the category of "Other Health Impairment" (OHI), and in the 2013–2014 school year that number rose to 817,000! Children categorized as OHI often carry a medical diagnosis such as diabetes or a mental health diagnosis such as anxiety that is so severe they require special educational programming.

What is perhaps more interesting about these statistics is that the percentage of students receiving services for physical/structural-based disabilities such a visual or speech impairment stayed essentially the same from 1977 through 2013, at 0.1 percent and 2.9 percent, respectively, yet the number of students with brain-based disabilities has skyrocketed.[40]

Self-Regulation Challenges

One of the greatest threats to learning we've observed is the large number of students who lack the ability to self regulate. We are seeing self-regulation difficulties in many children, not just those diagnosed with a learning disability, so this is an issue in the classroom that is not even included in all the statistics we have already provided! Self-regulation includes the ability to:

- Sustain attention

- Inhibit impulsivity

- Delay gratification

- Regulate emotions

- Complete tasks

- Cope and persevere when things are challenging

A recent study replicated a study of self-regulation first performed in the late 1940s, in which psychological researchers asked kids ages 3, 5, and 7 to stand perfectly still without moving. In the 1940s' experiment, the 3-year-olds couldn't stand still at all, the 5-year-olds could do it for about three minutes, and the 7-year-olds could stand pretty much as long as the researchers asked.

In 2001, researchers repeated this experiment, but psychologist Elena Bodrova at the National Institute for Early Education

Research says the results were very different. "Today's 5-year-olds were acting at the level of 3-year-olds 60 years ago, and today's 7-year-olds were barely approaching the level of a 5-year-old 60 years ago," Bodrova explains. "So the results were very sad." To be clear, the 5-year-olds could not stand still, and this reflects a real and quantifiable difference in the ability of children to self-regulate.

Another study conducted in the 1960s and 1970s at Stanford University by Walter Mischel found that the longer children delayed gratification, the better they would fare later in life at numerous measures of what we now call *executive function* (more on that in chapter 2). They would perform better academically, earn more money, and overall be healthier and happier. They would also be more likely to avoid a number of negative outcomes, including jail time, obesity, and drug use.

In the study, young children were given the option of eating a marshmallow right away or waiting. If they could wait, they would be given a second marshmallow. Of course, some little ones ate the marshmallow right away. Others looked at it, licked it, and literally spun themselves around in a chair to keep from eating it, so they could have a second. Mischel followed those children for the next five decades and found a positive trajectory for those who waited for the second marshmallow. As Roy Baumeister, a professor of psychology specializing in the study of willpower at Florida State University, says, "Self-control is like a muscle: the more you use it, the stronger it gets. Avoiding something tempting once will help you develop the ability to resist other temptations in the future."[41]

Declining Success in College

In the last decade, on average, 3.3 million students graduated from high school annually. In 2013, the National Center for Education reported that 65.9 percent of high school graduates went directly on to college. However, "Pathways to Prosperity," a Harvard Graduate School of Education study published in 2011, showed that only 56 percent of students who began a four-year degree finished it within six years.[42]

The Organization for Economic Co-operation and Development studied 18 countries, and the United States came in last for preparing its students for college readiness, with 46 percent of the students who started a degree (either two or four year) ever finishing it.[43]

In their article, "America Desperately Needs to Redefine College and Career Ready," Ted Dintersmith and Tony Wagner confirmed that in 2016 the percentage of students graduating college was just a bit over 50 percent, and that only half of those graduates landed jobs that paid well enough to justify the expenditure of college. These are disappointing facts that echo the findings of the Harvard study; American students are ill prepared for college and life success.[44]

Government programs, like those we discussed in the introduction, have been policing educational practice and instruction for nearly two decades, yet in the United States the majority of students who start a college degree program either do not finish it or cannot finish it in four years. Perhaps, curriculum and instruction and the way it is all implemented are not the reason for the declining performance of our children.

We would like to be clear that we have observed a general decline in the ability of *all* students, not just those who go off to college. We have also noticed a decline in a student's ability to perform tasks that were once done with ease, and not just in those students who are identified with a learning disability. We will share anecdotes and personal observations that back up our claims throughout the book, but we also thought it important to share data that validates our thoughts and claims.

The Takeaway

When you add together the number of children who are diagnosed with asthma, allergies, ADHD, and autism, it comes to 20 million children. In other words, one-third or more of all American children are challenged by the effects of these diagnoses, with some being life threatening. This does not include all the other children who are struggling with skills like self-regulation but carry no diagnosis. We think it is fair to say that children today are facing challenges, and that these more generalized learning and health issues are the elephant in the classroom that the federal government is not addressing. We urge you not to wait until the government steps in, as we can all be a part of changing some of these things now. By learning about the potential underlying causes of these rising rates, you can develop an action plan for your family and you may be able to minimize the impact on your children.

Chapter two

How the Brain Works

"Neuroplasticity provides us with a brain that can adapt not only to changes inflicted by damage, but allows adaptation to any and all experiences and changes we may encounter."

— HealingTraumaCenter.com

Think of a time when you had to rely on someone to tell you about something that you didn't understand for yourself. It could have been the mechanic or an appliance or computer repair person. If the news of a repair came with a hefty price tag, you might have felt even more anxious, wondering if what you were being told was true. Was everything that was recommended necessary? Imagine that you already had a basic understanding of mechanics or operating systems. That would enable you to ask some questions that would provide further clarification and understanding, and you would feel a sense of empowerment. This is how we want you to feel about your children and how they "operate" and learn. If you have a basic understanding of the brain and how it communicates with the body, you can make better sense of information that your pediatrician or your child's teachers are telling you. You may not have a complete understanding of how the brain works, but you can have enough information to determine where you need to learn more. The goal of this chapter is to lay a foundation that will help you make sense of how your child learns and feels, so that if you have concerns, or if a professional is sharing some concerns with you, you won't feel like you are in the dark.

The Brain: It's Plastic!

While science has revealed much about the human brain and body in the last few decades, the information has been very slow to make its way to the field of education and traditional medicine where teachers and doctors could use it to educate parents. Here, we attempt to get everyone on the same page.

First, we want to address our use of the words *plastic* and *plasticity*, as these words will be used throughout the chapter and the book. Neuroplasticity, as used in the fields of medicine and neuroscience, refers to the brain's ability to change for better or worse by forming new neural connections all throughout an individual's lifespan. The brain responds to positive and negative experiences such as meditation, exercise, new experiences, learning, diet, emotions, social interactions, paying attention, stress, and traumatic events. Neuroplasticity allows the brain to compensate for negative experiences such as injury, disease, and inflammation, and respond to positive interventions, situations, or environmental stimulation. That said, a negative experience is five times more likely to have a harmful impact on the brain than a positive one. Therefore, our efforts should be aimed at eliminating negativity in thought, word or deed, and where possible, we should bolster the brain through positive experiences and reinforcement.[1] The great news of neuroplasticity is that we don't necessarily have to accept whatever brain we are born with!

In order to understand the hope that neuroplasticity brings, you must first have a general understanding of how the brain works. If some of this information feels very new or overwhelming, just read through it once to get a sense for the big picture; we recommend circling back around and rereading this again once you have read other chapters. Soon you will learn that certain behaviors and different learning disabilities can be traced to malfunction in specific parts of the brain, and that some of the revolutionary therapies and interventions highlighted in this book work directly on or with those parts of the brain to achieve biological and behavioral improvements.

The Brain and Nervous System 101

The brain is divided into three basic parts: the forebrain, midbrain, and hindbrain. The brain develops in a relatively orderly sequence from back to front, with circuits that process lower-level information maturing before those that process higher-level thinking. The hindbrain includes the spinal cord and the brain stem and a small ball of tissue called the cerebellum, which regulates things like breathing, movement, balance, and heart rate. The midbrain controls some reflex actions, eye movement, and other voluntary actions. The forebrain is the largest, most visible, and highly developed part of the brain and is mostly composed of something called the cerebrum. The cerebrum is split into two halves, known as the right and left hemispheres, and though they look quite alike, they actually house very different functions. The two hemispheres are connected by a thick tract of nerves called the corpus callosum, which allows for communication between both sides.

Within the two hemispheres are structures called the frontal, parietal, occipital, temporal, and limbic lobes, each responsible for specific functions (figure 2.1). The brain contains billions of nerve cells known as neurons, which transmit information throughout the body's nervous system.[2]

The nervous system is divided into two parts. It includes the central nervous system, which is located in the brain and spinal cord and was originally thought to be hardwired at birth, and the peripheral nervous system, which contains a complex system that brings messages from the body's sense receptors to the brain and spinal cord and then carries messages from the brain and spinal cord to the muscles and glands throughout the body. The nervous system contains neurons, the same kind found in the brain, which can receive either excitatory or inhibitory signals. In other words, they receive messages that cause them to do more of something (excitatory) or less (inhibiting). A neurotransmitter is the chemical messenger that delivers information between neurons.[3]

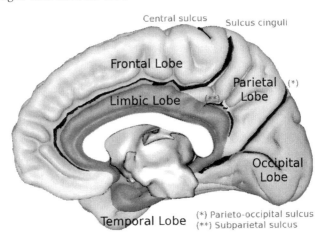

Figure 2.1 Lobes of the brain

The peripheral nervous system was always believed to be plastic, or capable of changing. As an example of how this was first understood, just think about stroke victims who lose the ability to use their right arm but then learn how to use their left instead, or amputees who lose a body part but learn that another part can be trained to compensate for the function of the lost part. The brain and body must be able to change, otherwise those adaptations couldn't happen. Science has now also proven that the central nervous system is capable of change and adaptation.[4] This gives great hope to children and adults who have issues within that system because therapies exist and more are being developed to work with the plasticity of this system.

The Brain as a House

Dr. Dan Siegel and Dr. Tina Payne Bryson offer a great analogy for thinking about brain functions and structure. If you envision the brain as a two-story house, the downstairs is where important things are located. In a house, it's where we find the kitchen, living room, and bathroom. In the brain, it's the part that is with us when we are born and never leaves us. It houses automatic responses necessary to life, such as breathing, heart rate, and innate reactions to danger (such as the fight, flight, or freeze response). The upstairs brain is more complex. We use the upstairs brain to think critically, problem solve, and make decisions. The whole upstairs brain, like the frontal lobe, is not fully formed until our mid-20s, which is something to consider when working with teens and young adults![5]

A Brief History of Brain Research

Researchers, doctors, and neuroscientists began mapping the brain in the 1930s. In the 1960s and 1970s, this kind of work was carried on by Robert Merzenich, who through a series of groundbreaking experiments, proved the brain was plastic, or changeable throughout all of life. A brain map represents an area of the brain where specific neurons and neuronal pathways can be traced to specific functions. For example, certain areas of the brain are responsible for seeing or hearing.[6]

As more and more research was carried out, scientists began naming areas of the brain within the lobes and the abilities housed within them. For example, Broca's area is a bundle of neurons in the frontal cortex behind the left eye that is involved in speech, and it helps us put our thoughts into words.[7] A study done by MIT and Boston

Children's Hospital showed that there is an abnormality in the brain scans of children with dyslexia connecting Broca's area to another area called Wernicke's area. In the future, a scan may be used to help with earlier identification of dyslexia.[8] Another area of the brain is the amygdala, which is an almond-shaped structure located deep in the brain's temporal lobe. The amygdala is involved in the storage of memories, and it is also thought to play a significant role in our experience of fear. Scientists are currently busy at work studying whether there could be neurotransmitter imbalances in the amygdala that may play a role in anxiety-based conditions like obsessive-compulsive disorder (OCD) and posttraumatic stress disorder (PTSD).[9] There will be more on neurotransmitters later in the chapter.

Modern Science and Neuroimaging

While the early work on brain research involved invasively investigating the brain through many different kinds of experiments, nowadays scientists, doctors, and researchers can get a look at the brain through noninvasive means. For example a SPECT scan, a type of nuclear imaging test, uses a radioactive substance and special camera to create three-dimensional images. Whereas an X-ray can show what your body's structures look like, a SPECT scan can show how your organs are working. In the case of looking at brain disorders, a scan can be helpful in pinpointing what parts of the brain are possibly being affected by dementia, clogged blood vessels, seizures, epilepsy, and head injuries. Images from your scan may show colors that help your doctor to identify areas where brain cells are less active versus more active; it can show if the brain is functioning typically, if it is inflamed, and can identify areas of the brain that were affected by injury or trauma. Many people forget about past injuries, especially if they occurred in childhood; however, these injuries can have long-term consequences on brain health.[10] Because many cognitive functions are now linked to specific areas of the brain, a SPECT scan can be a useful tool in pinpointing the areas of the brain involved in behavioral, emotional, or cognitive struggles, and these scans are actually being used by some rehab centers throughout the country. Other noninvasive brain imaging tools include magnetic resonance imaging (MRI), functional MRI (fMRI), computed tomography scans (also referred to as CT or CAT scans), and electroencephalography (EEG).

Fun Brain Facts

- The right hemisphere of the brain houses the nonverbal abilities, including the ability to read visual cues and body language. We tell children that the "right side of the brain likes working with pictures."

- The left hemisphere of the brain houses more of the verbal functions (though some skills related to speech are located on the right side). We tell children that the "left side of the brain likes working with words."

- The two hemispheres work independently of each other until about the age of 5 or 6. They have to "talk" to each other for true reading to occur. This is why, for most children, you cannot force the skill of reading any earlier. Simply put, one side likes reading the words, and the other side likes visualizing the concept like "making a movie in your mind," which is what reading is all about!

- The frontal lobe houses something known as executive function skills, including planning, organizing, regulating and sustaining attention, task initiation, inhibiting impulsivity, regulating emotions, sustaining effort and processing speed, accessing recall and working memory, cognitive flexibility, and problem solving. This is the last area to develop, often not reaching maturity until the mid to late 20s, and it is the first area of the brain to decline with old age. It is extremely important to recognize that this brain development continues into the 20s, and this is why we cannot expect children and teenagers to make decisions like adults do.

- The parietal lobe houses the mechanisms that give us information on taste, smell, touch, and temperature.

- The occipital lobe processes information taken in by the eyes in the form of light and other visual cues and links that information to stored memories. This is where words are stored for automatic access when reading and writing.

- The temporal lobe processes information taken in by the ears.

- The limbic lobe is located deeper in the brain and is part of the limbic system. It has several key functions due to its strategic location and connections with the rest of the brain. It is involved in the sense of smell, decision-making, motivation, expression of emotions, and memory. The reward, pleasure, and addiction center of the brain is also housed here.[11]

Many people are familiar with the idea of the left and right brain, and even sometimes refer to themselves as more of a left- or right-brained individual. The popular notion is that the left side of the brain houses things like logic, math, language, and words, and that "left-brain" people are more analytical; the right side of the brain houses things like intuition, the imagination, feelings, and the ability to visualize things as images, thus the "right-brain" person is considered to be more creative. While there may be some truth to this idea, the fact is that the brain is not that black and white. In reality, the two sides of the brain work together to process information, and modern research on this topic continues to validate this point.

Windows of Opportunity: Brain Growth and Learning

Although brain development can be enhanced by environmental experiences, it generally cannot be rushed. This is why you can't train a newborn to walk or talk, as those brain structures just aren't developed yet. Yet, there are "sensitive periods" when certain brain areas are primed for development. Young children need exposure to the right stimuli during these sensitive periods, otherwise certain neuronal circuits may not develop to their potential. The premise of "use it or lose it" applies to the brain. If pathways and connections aren't established during their sensitive periods, they will eventually be pruned (cut back) away by a special kind of white blood cell called microglia.[12,13] So while these windows of opportunity don't generally slam shut completely, learning at a later age will never be as easy as it would have been during these sensitive periods.

Pruning does not occur haphazardly. It depends largely on how any one brain pathway is used. If an activity is done frequently, the neural pathways involved in that activity are reinforced and deeply established. In contrast, if we do a task infrequently, the weak neural pathways will not be reinforced. The brain, being the amazing thing that it is, cuts off unused pathways; it will become more efficient for the person it belongs to. In other words, our brains are shaped largely in response to the demands we place on them.

This concept of pruning is very important for parents to understand. In order for the brain to develop properly, infants, toddlers, and children must physically engage with and explore their world. It is important for children to engage in a myriad of activities because this increases their opportunities to develop and diversify their skills. For this reason, it is also imperative that parents encourage their children to engage in activities that are difficult for them (remaining mindful of tasks that are developmentally appropriate for them to be engaging in, of course). Avoiding tasks that are difficult, whether they be physical or learning oriented in nature may hinder the opportunity to build stronger neural pathways related to skill-building. Many well-meaning parents decide that rather than watch their child struggle, they prefer to create scenarios that help them avoid difficulties or more easily succeed. While it is great to be helpful, being too helpful can come with a cost; helping your child avoid challenges may ultimately limit the extent to which certain neural pathways develop.

If your child is struggling to learn or accomplish something, consider finding a qualified professional who can work with your child and/or show you how to break the learning of the task down into smaller parts and then slowly build up the skill. Sometimes this means just working on something 5 minutes a day when you'd really love to spend more like 30 minutes. However, doing the task repeatedly, even in small chunks daily or several times a week, slowly reinforces those weak pathways, so something is happening, even if you don't see the gains right away. Oftentimes, parents can figure out ways to break down physical or learning tasks into smaller more manageable chunks; however, if your child is still struggling, there could be a greater issue at play, such as some weaknesses in executive function or motor planning. In chapter 10, we discuss several therapies and interventions that can help in this regard.

We'd like to clarify that the idea of use it or lose it applies to all children, not just those with an identified physical or learning challenge. Many children have strengths and weaknesses in their ability to learn certain subjects or have an unusually strong talent, whether that is an affinity for sports or the fine arts. While it is natural to celebrate the things that come easy, we have seen many parents allow children to focus a lot more on the area(s) of strength than on the area(s) of weakness. Yet, from what we know of the brain, children need to learn to spend more time on their weaknesses, too. We encourage parents to think about the long term, as we have seen scenarios such as a child putting aside academics to focus on a college or professional career in a sport only to suffer a devastating injury or burn out at some point. We've also seen some students push challenging courses like higher-level math to the side early in high school only to decide later that they aspire to be an engineer, and now they must play catch up to meet course requirements in college.

In case you are feeling discouraged that your child may have missed critical windows of opportunity, do not stress—there is hope! While there are times when the development of specific functions are optimized (for example, language development is optimal from birth through age 8), studies show us that with the right opportunities and exposure the brain can continue to develop and become more refined and better at cognitive functions throughout our lives, not just during these windows in the womb and in early infancy and childhood.[14] Consider that there are plenty of adults who are still able to learn a new language; yes, it's true that the younger you are the easier it seems to learn quickly, but we can learn a new language later in life. Learning later in life simply takes some extra, strategic effort.

The Brain and Multitasking

We know that the more you repeat and use a skill, the more that part of the brain develops, and the more you practice a skill, the faster you become at performing that skill. However, remember Robert Merzenich and his work on brain mapping mentioned earlier in the chapter? His research showed that neural pathways and the brain mapping attached to a given task only strengthens when there is sustained attention to that specific task. That means that when attention is divided, the pathway weakens.[15] In understanding this fact, it is easy to see how the learning of a child with attentional problems can sometimes suffer. Also, we live in a world where people are multitasking all the time, yet the research suggests the strength and the intelligence of the brain decline while multitasking. As educators, one of the greatest detriments to learning that we see is a student studying with the distraction of devices. Trying to type a report on the computer or comprehend information in a textbook while going in and out of Facebook or Twitter, cannot lead to optimal performance or absorption of material. Or, consider the more dangerous trend of adults and teenagers driving while either talking on the phone or texting. While people may believe they can do all things well at the same time, brain maps tell us otherwise.

Chemical Composition of the Brain

During the same period of great brain research when scientists were mapping the physical structures of the brain, others were discovering the brain's chemical composition. For example, it was learned that neurons communicate amongst themselves by releasing chemical messengers, known as neurotransmitters, in the spaces between neurons called the synaptic cleft (figure 2.2).[16]

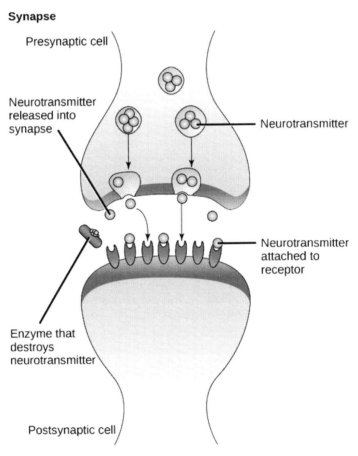

Synapse

Presynaptic cell

Neurotransmitter released into synapse

Neurotransmitter

Neurotransmitter attached to receptor

Enzyme that destroys neurotransmitter

Postsynaptic cell

Figure 2.2 Synapse

The Chemical Messengers

Serotonin is often referred to as the "mood" neurotransmitter and can be found primarily in the digestive system, although it can be in blood platelets and throughout the central nervous system, too. It plays a vital role in emotional health from positive emotions of happiness to not-so-great feelings of anxiety and depression. It helps decrease our worries and concerns and is also tied to other biological processes, including attention, sleep, appetite, digestion, and healing of wounds. Sometimes, without knowing a neurotransmitter imbalance can be at play, people who are low in serotonin can crave simple carbs, "white" foods or "mood foods" such as breads, muffins, cereals, pasta, and foods containing sugar. Consuming these foods causes a spike in insulin that helps people feel more relaxed and less worried for the time being; in other words, they feel happy. Then, as blood sugar levels drop, they may experience "brain fog" or feel "hangry" (hungry-angry) again and crave those same foods. It's a vicious cycle, and it may lead people to become dependent or even addicted to these types of foods. Brain-healthy foods that boost serotonin include protein rich foods such as eggs, tofu, salmon, turkey, red meats, cheese, nuts, and seeds.[17,18]

Dopamine is a neurotransmitter that plays a role in attention, memory, motivation, and motor skills. It is also involved in the reward and pleasure centers of the brain and is the neurotransmitter that helps you get things done. Low levels of dopamine lead to attention problems and, if severe enough, potentially to a diagnosis such as attention deficit disorder (ADD). Low levels of dopamine can also lead to issues with regulating attention and focus, lack of motivation, time and materials management, and impulse control, all problems teachers see in many of their students. Low levels are also now being discovered as part of the shaking/tremors a person with Parkinson's experiences. High levels are associated with a state of "mania" and can even lead to delusions.[19] Foods that help boost dopamine levels include poultry, fish, eggs, seeds, cheese, apples, bananas, beets, kale, strawberries, blueberries, and green tea.[20]

Epinephrine (also known as adrenaline) regulates attention, focus, and cognition. High amounts have been linked to hyperactivity, sleep problems, and anxiety. (Imagine what it would feel like if you had too much adrenaline pumping through your blood.) Deficient amounts lead to lack of focus, fatigue, and difficulty losing weight.

Norepinephrine (also known as noradrenaline) modulates many other cell and brain functions. It is responsible for picking up the signals that can cause your body to go into that "fight-or-flight" mode, the system that allows your body to know that it is in danger. If you have an excessive amount of this neurotransmitter, your body might always feel like it is fighting off some danger. Hypervigilance and ultimately exhaustion are the result.

Acetylcholine was the first discovered neurotransmitter. It plays a critical role in the formation of memories and verbal and logical reasoning. Diminishing amounts have been tied to conditions such as Alzheimer's.

GABA is the major calming or inhibitory neurotransmitter. In a sense, it is nature's "sedative." GABA helps neurons recover after they fire, hence reducing anxiety, worry, and fear. When GABA is low or depleted, you can expect to see more anxiety, worry, and sleep disturbance.

Neurotransmitters are found in the brain, immune system, gut, and the glands and are supposed to be present in very specific amounts. Therefore, even small imbalances in neurotransmitters can cause dysfunction in the brain and body. It is also now known that genetic mutations can change the regulation of neurotransmitters, leading to a lack of or too much of one or more neurotransmitter. Chronic stress, poor nutrition, poor sleep, and general inflammation, all problems many adults and children struggle with, can cause the neurotransmitters to lose proper balance.[21]

Miscommunicated Messages

While this is an overly simplistic explanation of a complex brain function, you can think of neurotransmitter communication like the popular childhood game "whisper down the lane." A neuron picks up a message or signal and then passes it off to the next neuron via neurotransmitters in the synaptic cleft, and then this process between neurons and neurotransmitters is repeated until the message reaches its intended destination.

Information can come from many sources. For example, when a hand touches something hot, the sense receptors in the skin feel the heat, then deliver a message via neural circuits and neurotransmitters to the brain: "When I touch the oven, it is hot!" Now imagine that you had an imbalance of neurotransmitters. Let's say you have too much epinephrine, the fight-or-flight neurotransmitter. So now when you go near the oven and feel the heat, your neurons are overexcitedly delivering the message about the heat, and you have an over-the-top reaction (and everyone around you is wondering what the dramatic response is all about). It should at least be considered that a neurotransmitter imbalance could be the cause of extreme behaviors.

Parents tend to feel relieved once they understand that there may be a real biological reason why their child is struggling or exhibiting behaviors that don't make sense. Oftentimes parents blame themselves if their child is having problems, or they feel angry and disappointed with their child because they interpret their child's behavior as willful or disobedient. We want to shift energy away from blame, anger, sadness and frustration and toward finding the underlying cause of whatever the issue may be. In chapter 10, we offer information about how an integrative medical doctor or psychiatrist might run tests to look at neurotransmitter levels.

Brain Science Applied to Learning

A relatively recent discovery related to brain mapping revealed insight on children with language-based disabilities, a kind of disability that an estimated 5 percent to 10 percent of children have. It was found that children with language-based disabilities often have auditory processing problems, meaning they can hear sound but are not interpreting it correctly within the brain. Researchers were frustrated because though they could "describe" the problem these children faced, they had no solution. It was hypothesized that the neurons involved in the auditory process were likely not firing fast enough for the child to keep up while trying to listen, and hence was missing a lot of valuable auditory information. Research on brain mapping showed that neurons, after they have fired off following a round of auditory information, required about 30 milliseconds to refire. However, the neurons of 80 percent of the children with language-based impairments took at least three times as long.[22] When a child doesn't hear information presented in the classroom correctly, it sets off a cascade effect that impairs all other kinds of learning. Based on this hypothesis, the program Fast ForWord® was born, and it has been successful in correcting this problem. Of 500 children enrolled in a study of Fast ForWord®, the average child moved 1.8 years ahead in language development after only six weeks on the program.[23] As educators, we can tell you—this is remarkable! And of course, Fast ForWord® has been adapted to address other kinds of learning-based disabilities.[24] You can learn more about Fast ForWord® in chapter 10.

Many children also struggle with reading. The first key thing to know about reading difficulties is that they are rarely related to IQ or natural intelligence. Some children just need more time and exposure to reading instruction, whereas others continue to struggle despite reading tutoring and reading support in school. Teachers are often mystified, and parents' stamina and patience are put to the test when trying to help their child practice this skill. These children seem to have a "word blindness" and don't naturally process the written word. So why can't they learn to read?

Researchers have studied what they call "dyslexic brains" and have found that two areas in the left hemisphere are underactivated. The first area is the left temporoparietal cortex, which is typically the first area of the brain to be used to process spoken language and begin to sound out words. For example, your child sees "cat" and says /c/ /a/ /t/ and blends the sounds together to say and read "cat." Then, hopefully, your child begins to automatically recognize the word "cat," or better yet, any word that has the "at" pattern and is able to fluently read fat, mat, that, sat, etc. Many students have a weakness in this reading skill, and excellent reading programs, such as Wilson Reading, Fundations, and Project READ, have successfully taught students who have this type of reading difficulty to become successful readers. However, if a child is constantly struggling to read "cat" and has to sound it out every time he or she sees it, as if seeing it for the first time, then it is possible there is something else going on.

We learned that the second area of the left hemisphere, the occipitotemporal cortex, is underactivated in some children, and this area, located at the base of the brain behind our ears, is the visual processing center of our brains. Prior to learning to read, this part of the brain recognizes common objects—a fork, a chair, eyeglasses, etc. No matter which way we look at those objects, they will always be the same to us. (This is not the case with the letters b, d, p, q, m, u, and w, because when rotated a certain way they will be perceived as completely different letters.) As we become readers, we train this area of the brain to visually recognize letters, phonetic patterns, and common sight words. For children to become fluent and automatic readers and spellers, they need both the left temporoparietal cortex and occipitotemporal cortex to be activated and working efficiently.[25] The question then becomes how do we activate those areas, specifically the one that allows for automatic word recognition (the occipitotemporal cortex)? The good news is that there are ways and specific programs that retrain the brain to be able to visualize and remember symbols and words. If "making a movie" is hard (right hemisphere task), there is help for that, too. The programs to look for in chapter 10 are Lindamood Bell's Seeing Stars and Visualization and Verbalization.

As we have shared, so much is now known about neurons, neurotransmitters, and neural networks and their roles in learning, behavior, and mental and physical health, and some doctors are using this knowledge to treat mental and physical health issues. Even some educators in some schools are beginning to educate students and staff about brain development.

The Brain–Body Connection: It's Electric!

The brain and the rest of the body are in constant communication. We have already talked a bit about neurons and neurotransmitters, the chemical messengers. Now, believe it or not, we'd like to share that some of the other information transmitted throughout the body is delivered via signals that are electric and magnetic in nature. Through the use of highly sensitive equipment, researchers have been able to detect these signals and therefore prove what were once just theories and speculation about this brain–body communication.

If you've ever witnessed a scene unfold of someone having a heart attack on your favorite medically oriented television show, you've seen how the doctors use a system that includes electrically charged paddles, called a defibrillator, to jumpstart the heart back into a regular beating pattern. They use electrically charged paddles because the heart contains cells that generate electrical activity all on their own, and these cells cause the heart to contract rhythmically, making a heartbeat. These cells are called pacemaker cells, and they cause the heart to contract more than once per second, leading to a "normal" heart rate of 72 beats per minute.[26] It was later discovered that other cells in the body produce electrical activity, including neurons and muscle cells. This electric activity creates a magnetic field surrounding the body. In fact, "brain waves," or brain activity, are not confined to the brain but actually spread throughout the body via the nervous system.[27]

Research carried out at the Heart Math Institute reveals that in addition to the extensive neural communication network linking the heart with the brain and body, the heart also communicates information to the brain and throughout the body via electromagnetic field interactions. The continuous communication between the heart and brain influences the brain's perception, cognition, and emotional processing.

Science has shown us that the experiences and reactions of the brain and the body emanate from the body via this magnetic and electrical system. Therefore, our reactions are not actually contained within our own body but spread beyond our body. This fact was actually captured on film by New York Times bestselling author Dr. Masaru Emoto. In his book, *The Hidden Messages in Water*, Emoto shares numerous photographs of the crystals found in water and their physical changes in response to people who were expressing specific emotions within feet of the water. When children were reading positive messages aloud, the crystals had beautiful shapes. When monks were praying near the water, the crystals had intricate and delicate patterns. However, when people spoke angry and hateful words, the crystals would appear ugly and distorted.[28] This is important information because the average human body is 70 percent water. Every human cell and organ contains water, so if the way we are feeling impacts the water sitting in a glass next to us, it would stand to reason that the way we are feeling can have a profound impact on the health of the cells in our body.[29]

While the work of Dr. Emoto might seem fantastical, you will be pleased to know that there is a growing field of research at some of the most reputable institutions in America that support the conclusions Emoto drew from his photographic images. In fact, it has been shown that positive meditation (27 minutes a day for eight weeks) can produce "massive changes inside the brain's gray matter."[30] In other words, positive thoughts are able to literally change the physical structure of the brain!

It might also be of interest to you that the electrical energy of our bodies can interact with the environment. Did you ever notice you feel better by the ocean? Science has shown that spending time near the ocean can help us at the cellular level. Sea air and salt water contain negative ions that interact with the electric system within our body, accelerating our ability to absorb oxygen. The negative ions also balance serotonin, which if you remember, is a neurotransmitter that regulates mood and stress.[31] There are therapies within the field of medicine that are working with the body at the energetic and cellular level. Some of those therapies are highlighted in chapter 10.

So Why Does All of This Matter?

What we have learned is that our thoughts, feelings, and words impact our physical being, down to the composition of the very cells that make up our body. Understanding this should give us all reason to think more carefully about our thoughts, words, and feelings because they can literally impact our health and the health of others. We can use positive thoughts or exercises such as meditation to bolster ourselves and others. Conversely, we must also be mindful that as parents or others who care for children, our negative words said in anger or frustration can cause harm. Some schools and after school programs are working meditation and mindfulness into their programs; courses on yoga, meditation, and mindfulness for kids and teens are available in many communities; and parents can also teach their kids meditation and the power of positive thinking at home!

Chapter three

Milestones From Infancy Through Late Adolescence

"Within the child lies the fate of the future."

—Maria Montessori

The happiness, well-being, and education of our children are each influenced by a number of factors. While the focus of this book is on how some of these key factors impact a child's ability to learn and thrive in life and in school, we argue that the experience of "school" starts long before formal schooling ever takes place and is based on more than instruction from classroom teachers. Parents play a critical role in the early development of their children, and yet it's the one job for which there is no formal training. It is our hope that the information contained in this chapter will provide a basic understanding of child development.

Understanding the milestones of child development helps people understand what the "norm," or average, is, knowing that the norm can be a broad band and is not an exact science. Nonetheless, developmental milestones can be used as a general guideline. Knowing what to expect at each stage can be a comfort to parents, and having an understanding of whether your child's development is on or off track can allow you to seek help earlier if you have concerns.

The Center on the Developing Child at Harvard University states, "Decades of rigorous research show that children's earliest experiences play a critical role in brain development. The brain is most 'plastic' or flexible during the first three years of life. High quality, early intervention services can change a child's developmental trajectory and improve outcomes for children, families and communities." They also point out that, "Intervention is likely to be more effective and less costly when it is provided earlier in life rather than later." We feel that if more parents were armed with adequate developmental information, that in many instances they may be able to head off the need for early intervention.[1]

Clearly, early intervention is beneficial when it can or does happen. However, if your children are well into their childhood, it is still worth it to understand the principles in this chapter because you can go back and work on things that were not achieved earlier and build upon them. Remember, the brain continues to grow and develop throughout life, and given certain interventions it can build and establish new pathways and become capable of functions it couldn't do before. Many different therapies and interventions have shown great success at changing and improving brain and cognitive function at all ages. We highlight many of these strategies in chapter 10.

Each child is unique and will develop and master skills at his or her own rate, though normally this will still fall within a certain time frame of development. It is not unusual for a child to be advanced in one area while developing at a slower rate in another area. Just like adults, children have natural likes and dislikes, and so they will spend more time working on things that they enjoy, though it is important for parents to try to help them build skills in the child's less desired areas.

Another reason that it is important for parents to understand the developmental stages their child goes through is so that they understand that the body and brain develop in a specific way and at specific times, so we must be mindful to not place certain expectations on children before they are truly ready to meet them. While many children develop skills and capabilities within a set time, some children can be late bloomers, and sometimes just need the gift of extra time. This may come in the form of an extra year of preschool if the child has a late spring or summer birthday, or it might look like a transitional pre-first grade year between kindergarten and first grade in schools that offer this option. The key is to determine if the child just needs the cushion of a little extra time or whether something greater is going on that requires more specific attention.

Many books and online resources are available that provide parents with ideas about how to stimulate proper development, in addition to offering great detail about each area of child development and what to expect at various ages. Some of those resources will be listed at the end of this chapter.

The following information provides a general description of the different stages of development. This information was taken from a variety of sources, as well as from our own personal and professional experiences.

Birth to 2 Years[2,3,4]

Physical/Motor Development

Gross Motor Development

- Lifts head and chest when lying on stomach, kicks legs (3 months)
- Holds up head and rolls over (6 months)
- Begins to sits up with/without support (6 months)

- Creeps, crawls, cruises around furniture, maybe one to two steps (7 to 12 months)
- Walks independently (12 to 18 months)
- Kicks a ball, jumps, and runs (24 months)
- Climbs on furniture (24 months)

Fine Motor Development

- Explores objects with hands and mouth (7 months)
- Begins to pass things from one hand to another (7 months)
- Bangs two things together (12 months)
- Puts things in a container (12 months)
- Finds hidden things (12 months)
- Uses spoon and fork (12 to 18 months)
- Uses a cup (12 to 18 months)
- Makes or copies a straight line or circle (24 months)
- Builds towers of four or more blocks (24 months)

Language Development

Receptive Language

- Begins to babble and to imitate some sounds (3 months)
- Smiles when hears parents' voices (3 months)
- Enjoys playing with other people (3 months)
- Makes eye contact and social smile (3 months)
- Responds to sounds and to their own name (6 months)
- Responds to "no" (12 months)

- Can point to pictures, body parts, or people by name (24 months)

- Follows simple instructions (24 months)

Expressive Language

- Cries to express discomfort or when needs are not being met (their cries will change and it will become easier to distinguish the reason for crying) (0 to 24 months)

- Stringing vowel sounds together and beginning to say consonant sounds (6 months)

- May say "mama," "dada," or "uh oh" (12 months)

- Says several words (18 months)

- Repeats words heard in conversation (24 months)

- Can speak in two- to four-word sentences (24 months)

- May have up to 50 words (24 months)

Social/Emotional Development

- Will develop a sense of trust or mistrust that basic needs will be met (i.e., adequate food, clothing, shelter, and response to emotional needs)

- Knows familiar faces and begins to recognize if someone is a stranger (6 months)

- May experience separation anxiety and stranger anxiety (seems to reach a peak between 10 to 18 months)

- Begins and enjoys playing games like "peek-a-boo" and "pat-a-cake" (7 to 12 months)

- Understands emotions by tone of voice (7 months)

- Has developed favorite things and people (12 months)

- Begins to play make believe (24 months)

- Wants to do things on their own (24 months)

Cognitive Development

- Learns by exploring with hands and mouth (3 to 24 months)

- Tries to imitate behaviors that are observed (i.e., simple cleaning tasks) (12 months)

- Finds hidden objects (12 months)

- Hands adult a book when he or she wants to hear a story (12 months)

- Follows simple directions (12 months)

- Begins to sort items by shapes and colors (24 months)

Summary

There is no greater time period of rapid and plentiful growth and change than from birth to age 2. It is so important for parents to dig deep within themselves to find the patience to allow their children to learn from their mistakes and develop a sense of autonomy. There will be a lot of spilled milk and messes to clean up together during this time, but understand that the ultimate goal is for children to feel a sense of accomplishment and security in the idea that they can take care of their own basic needs. Another major stressor during this phase of development is separation anxiety. Again, it is normal for children to feel anxious but important for parents to allow periods of separation (this may need to be done more slowly for some children) so that children understand that it will be okay when a parent is not with them. It will also help children learn to reach out to and communicate with other caring adults in preparation for going to school one day.

As this phase comes to an end, you will be entering the world known as the "terrible twos." We would encourage you to reframe your mindset and not look at this as a bad period of time, but rather a time to find your sense of humor and really appreciate what is really happening below the surface. The window for developing emotional control starts around age 2. Remember the upstairs and downstairs brain from chapter 2: around age 2, there is an internal battle between the upstairs and downstairs brain. Children are trying to figure out whether a tantrum or a rational request will get them what they want and will frequently exhibit these types of conflicts. Parents beware—if tantrums often win out during this period, children will continue to use this strategy to get their way beyond age 2, and it will be very difficult to change this behavior later on. Some would say that a child's behavior at 2 is a good predictor of what the teenage years will be like.

Ages 3 to 5[5]

Physical/Motor Development

Physical

- Toilet trained (though some children will still need a pull-up at nighttime)

- Brushes teeth

- Dresses self, including buttoning, snapping, and zipping, but not always in the right order

- Shoelace tying is introduced but may not be mastered until ages 5 or 6

- Is establishing a hand dominance

- Tripod pencil grip may be emerging with coaching but not mastered by all 5-year-olds

Gross Motor Development

- Can balance

- Rides a trike

- Throws, catches, and bounces a ball

- Ascends and descends stairs with alternating feet

- Hops, climbs, and balances on one foot

- Tries many physical tasks and may become frustrated and experience mishaps

Fine Motor Development

- Cuts with scissors

- Copies shapes (i.e., circle, cross, rectangle, and square)

- Explores more fine motor opportunities with pencils, crayons, paints, scissors, crafts, lacing cards, etc.

- Can draw a person with up to four body parts

Language Development

Expressive Language Development

- Uses/understands up to 2,500 words

- Language is purposeful, more complex, and adult like

- Tells stories and uses descriptive words and language

- Strangers can understand speech

- Asks "why"

- Asks the meaning of words

Social/Emotional Development

- May play side by side in similar activities but still be playing separately, often called "parallel play"

- Begins to notice others, communicate, and share

- Cooperative play; works together with others for a common goal, and friendships begin to develop

- Imaginative and creative play; may have an imaginary friend

- Understands turn-taking

- Is learning to solve conflicts

- Feels pride in pleasing adults

- Increase in "testing the waters" by challenging parents

- Wants to understand "why"

- Has more control over range of emotion

- Compares actions to others; conformity to peers is important

- May not understand the difference between fantasy and reality, and therefore have nightmares or fear of monsters

- Makes independent choices

- Helps others and enjoys doing chores

- Better understanding of rules and right from wrong; begins to understand right from wrong and may feel a sense of shame for wrongdoing

- Increasing ability to pay attention despite distractions

Cognitive Development

Communication and Reading Readiness

- Answers questions about a story, rhyme, or song
- Is beginning to make predictions
- Identifies some letters
- Listens to and interacts with picture books and stories

Math

- Can count up to 10 objects
- Matches and sorts
- Recognizes and creates patterns
- Is beginning to understand concept of time (i.e., "in a minute," or "five-minute warning")

Other

- Knows his or her full name
- Names colors
- Identifies body parts
- Uses materials and tools to explore
- Is beginning to understand there is more than one solution to a problem

Summary

You may have noticed that the social/emotional component of this age group is quite lengthy. That is because this is a time where the skills involved in being able to understand the world from your own and differing perspectives is growing and is hopefully being modeled and nurtured by caring adults. Parents can encourage kindness, empathy, and understanding in their children by engaging in purposeful and rich discussions that will foster these characteristics. This could sound like the following:

- "How did you feel when your friend called you that name?"

- "How do you think the child who is alone on the playground is feeling? How might you help him?"

- "Wouldn't it be nice if you shared your new toy when your friend comes over to play?"

- "Do you think that Michael saw what happened differently than you did?"

- "Could you tell the teacher how you felt when you didn't understand the directions?"

- "When that didn't work, what else could you have tried?"

- "I am sorry that I yelled at you. Mommy is very tired, and it was wrong of me to become angry over something so silly. Will you please forgive me?"

- "Mommy and Daddy didn't handle that very well. Yelling and shouting don't help solve the problem. We will work harder to solve the problem differently next time."

Ages 6 to 11[6, 7]

Physical/Motor Development

Physical Development

- Losing baby teeth starts around age 5, most permanent teeth in by age 13
- Effectively performs grooming and eating tasks

Gross Motor Development

- Can ride a two-wheeler bike
- Skips, hops, jumps rope
- Likes and needs to move a lot
- Is gaining athletic skills and coordination
- Signs of puberty may be noticed

Fine Motor Development

Ages 6 to 8

- Learns how to hold a pencil correctly
- Learns how to print letters and write numerals
- Draws a triangle and diamond
- Draws a person with a head, body, and limbs
- Improves cutting skills

- Masters shoelace tying

- Uses computer/mouse (While we do not endorse encouraging more time spent on electronic devices, the reality is that the expectation in most schools today is that children have working knowledge of using a computer. We recommend nurturing overall fine motor skill development with strategies found in chapter 9.)

Ages 9 to 11

- Fine motor skills are perfected

- May or may not include cursive instruction, depending on school's curriculum

- Keyboarding skills are taught and improved

Language Development

Expressive Language Development

- Articulation of all speech sounds in place around the age of 8

- Intelligible speech

- Increasing use of correct grammar

Social/Emotional Development

Ages 6 to 8

- Prefers one to two friends

- Can be hard on younger siblings

- Tends to have their feelings easily hurt or to feel disappointed

- Still self-centered, may feel slighted if not getting attention
- Can have difficulty taking the perspective of others
- Capable of using good manners when prompted/taught
- Prefers structured activities to open-ended ones
- Great focus on rules for guiding behavior and activities
- May rely on adult approval
- Has a strong sense of following the rules
- Wants to feel competent or good at tasks attempted
- Develops greater awareness of social activities/roles such as romantic relationships and social behaviors such as swearing

Ages 9 to 11

- Enlarging circle of friends to three or four or more
- Play and peer interactions become less fantasy oriented and more oriented toward sports, games, and specific activities
- More competitive, and thus engages in more arguments and conflicts with peers
- Self-esteem very much tied to the mastery of social, physical, and academic tasks
- Begins to understand that some rules and social roles can be flexible; can adapt to the situation at hand
- Takes on more responsibilities at school and home
- Manners become more automatic (when they've been expected and reinforced)
- May experiment with social and romantic relationships (i.e., playing truth or dare with peers, hand holding or kissing, more engagement with social media)

Cognitive Development

Communication and Reading Readiness

Ages 6 to 8

- Reads with an emphasis on letters, sounds, decoding unknown words, sight word mastery (up to 400 words), and comprehension of text

- Spells common sight words and words with phonetic patterns

- Writes and shares stories

Ages 9 to 11

- Reads to learn with a focus on comprehension of fiction and nonfiction text

- More analytical and inferential thinking

- Spells common sight words and words with phonetic patterns

- Written expression is more mature

- Writing for purposes of information, directions (how to do something), persuasion, and creative expression

Math

Ages 6 to 8

- Concrete level of thinking

- Skip counting

- Place value
- Multiple strategies for computation of facts
- Addition and subtraction computation (up to four-digit numbers and multiple addends)
- Introduction of concept of multiplication
- Increased understanding of time and money
- Geometry/shapes
- Fractions
- Measurement

Ages 9 to 11

- Place value of whole numbers to millions
- Multiplication/division
- Graphing/tables/stem-and-leaf plots
- Mean, median, mode
- Angles (measure and draw)
- Lines (parallel, perpendicular, horizontal/vertical)
- Area/perimeter
- Symmetry
- Multiplying and dividing whole numbers
- Adding, subtracting, multiplying, and dividing fractions
- Adding, subtracting, multiplying, and dividing decimals
- Spatial reasoning and logic, which includes geometry and algebraic concepts
- Percentages
- Ratio/proportion
- Graphing and probability

Summary

Social and emotional development is still in full swing, and friendships are very important. The mid to later elementary years are when children begin to differentiate themselves from others based on interests and strengths, such as dolls, sports, music, academics, and Scouts. This may result in a change-up in friendships, and some children may feel the loss of former friendships more than others. It is important for parents to keep an eye on whether their children have friends. The number of friends is not important. It's the feeling of connectedness to at least one other child that matters. For some children, just having someone to sit with at lunch or play with at recess is enough to make their day feel emotionally safe and happy. Your school's guidance counselor can be a great resource for connecting kids and monitoring lunch and playground activities.

You may also have noticed that the cognitive/academic section has grown in length and detail during this period of development. This is because around age 7 the brain is undergoing a period of rapid and amazing growth, which includes a large blossoming of neurons. Educators take advantage of this time of rapid brain growth and increase academic demands. Remember back to the previous chapter on brain development, when brains are younger, they are more primed for learning. Teachers expose children to all kinds of educational material, hoping to engage the brain in as many ways as possible, and then they try to reinforce that learning by daily lessons and sometimes homework! Now what brain science shows us is that different neural pathways are being built by exposure to the different subject areas and then being more or less reinforced, depending on the amount of time the child studies or practices. When one looks at where children are upon entering kindergarten to where they are when leaving fifth grade, it is mind-boggling what has been accomplished during the elementary years.

There is an amazing "blossoming" of neurons that occurs around age 7. Synaptic or neural pruning intensifies after the rapid brain-cell proliferation during childhood and again in the period that encompasses adolescence and the 20s. Please keep this in mind as you read on and learn more about adolescent development.[8, 9]

Ages 12 to 14[10]

Physical/Motor Development

Physical Development

- Puberty
- Growth spurts can cause clumsiness
- Differences in development rates between boys and girls and within this age group in general
- Overly focuses on hygiene or avoids hygiene altogether
- Very aware of one's own sexuality
- Changes in sleeping patterns (preference for sleeping later in morning)

Gross Motor Development

- Athletic abilities blossom for some; this topic can be difficult for those who don't excel

Social/Emotional Development

- Enjoys the social aspect of learning
- Strong influence of friends and may prefer friends to parents/ family, may begin to distance self from parents in attempt to establish own identity

- Shift in circle of friends, cliques may form, peer pressure, very concerned with social acceptance

- Roller coaster of emotions, can be emotionally sensitive

- May be exposed to and/or choose to dabble in risky behaviors

- Self-conscious about physical appearance, especially in relationship to puberty/physical development

- Increasing fascination with different kinds of relationships and curiosity and possible experimentation in "romantic" relationships

Cognitive/Academic Development

- Moves from concrete to abstract thinking

- More analytical and critical-thinking ability

- Increase in problem-solving ability

- School-based instruction makes greater movement toward students being grouped by ability level within their grade

Summary

During this time, teens begin to separate from their parents and establish their own identity. Biologically they are doing so because soon they will be expected to achieve a level of independence from their parents. However, many parents really struggle with giving their child the space to do this because they are afraid that their child isn't ready to make mature decisions. Now we know that a lot is going on inside the brain during this tumultuous time.

Recall that the brain undergoes a period of significant remodeling during the adolescent years, which includes neural pruning. During the process of pruning, the brain is also laying down myelin sheaths, which protect the pathways that remain and allows them to communicate more quickly. The end result of this process is what scientists call "specialization." While the final product may be a more efficient brain, and one where the teen is able to identify and pursue his or her own strengths and interests, the brain is in fact under construction during this process. Specialization has been likened to the experience of doing a home renovation while living in the home. (For anyone who has done that, you know it is challenging!) When doing a renovation, there are messes and roadblocks to be worked around, causing frustration and requiring a deeper level of patience until the project is complete. However, once it is complete you can then enjoy the final product.[11] This is a potent analogy for parents. During all those changes in the adolescent brain, the teen may experience a reduction in executive function skills, such as impulse control, problem solving, attention, regulating emotional responses, and task initiation/completion. With a reduction in overall executive function skills, teens may not always consider the long-term consequences of their actions and may make some poor decisions.

Also of note is the real and increased need for sleep. Maybe you are a "morning person" and prefer to rise early, or perhaps you are a "night owl" and enjoy sleeping in longer in the morning. Most people do notice that they are more alert and sleepier at different times of the day. Our bodies have an internal clock of sorts called circadian rhythm that controls the body's natural sleep cycles. Everyone has daily peaks and valleys that are determined by exposure to daylight and other variables. The circadian rhythm dips and rises at different times of the day for different age groups. Think of young children who usually wake up very early in the morning and are in bed fairly early, and then think of adolescents who all of a sudden prefer to sleep until noon and stay up until all hours of the night! This is the perfect example of a normal shift in circadian rhythms. Preadolescents and adults are usually more alert from early morning until around noon or 1:00 p.m. and may feel like they need a nap in early afternoon. However, teens tend to lag behind by an hour or two.[12] They are not just being lazy in the morning or choosing to be a night owl after all; it is a natural shift in their circadian rhythm, which has caused the American Academy of Pediatrics to issue recommendations for a school start time of 8:30 a.m. or later for middle and high schools. Some school districts have adjusted the starting school time for those students, but many other schools around the country still start earlier.[13]

Ages 15 to 18[14]

Physical/Motor Development

Physical Development

- Puberty

- May look older than chronological age; maturation rates still vary

- Sleep cycles change, with teenagers preferring to sleep late

Social/Emotional Development

- May not want to spend a lot of time with parents, preferring to be with friends; may experience increased tension and conflicts as they begin to separate from parents, may ask friends for help before parents

- Emotional levels may vary (i.e., moodiness)

- May be exposed to and/or choose to dabble in risky behaviors

- More social and extracurricular activities are available

- Peer pressure is still an issue

- Examination of belief systems, wanting to understand their own beliefs as well as those of others, and friendships often become tied to common belief systems

- Dating and romantic relationships may become prioritized

Cognitive Development

- Expands logic and reasoning abilities

- Thinks hypothetically, draws conclusions

- Can expand thinking beyond the "black and white" and see shades of gray

- Has thoughtful discussions about many topics

- Talks/thinks about the future

- Can see the perspectives of others

- Can have more shared discussions with adults

Summary

There is no doubt that the teenage years can be trying times for parents, but try to focus on the fact that this struggle is a process teens must go through if they are to become independent adults. Of course there are absolutely times where a parent must step in because there is real danger, but other times we must risk letting them get a few bumps and bruises, or maybe more of a "bruised ego," as they make mistakes while they are busy "knowing it all." If we don't allow teens to make mistakes while they are still in the safety net of our home and where we can help them process mistakes after they happen, our teens will be ill equipped to manage life on their own after they leave the nest. Instead of yelling at or punishing your teen for a poor decision, sit down at the table and have a discussion, which might sound something like, "It looks like that didn't work out the way you had hoped for. Where do you think things went wrong? Do you have any ideas as to how it could go better the next time? If you are willing to hear me, I have some thoughts and ideas, too." By removing judgment and resisting the use of "I told you so," your teen will come to see that you really do want them to succeed and that you can be a great resource to them.

Speaking of bumps and bruises, adolescence is often a time where kids get more deeply involved in sports and other activities like learning to drive, and new drivers are more prone to accidents. If you recall, neural pruning is carried out by microglia cells. One of the amazing things about the brain is that after a head bump or trauma, those microglia cells kick in, and they prune out the damaged neurons. This sounds great, right? (Nature's own mechanism to heal and clean up the brain from injury!) It is great if the brain only had an occasional bump. However, as science has evolved and the brain is able to be studied more carefully, we are learning more about the frequent jarring that occurs when kids are tackled on the athletic fields, experience hard landings from falls during dance or gymnastic routines, or when they fall off bikes or playground equipment. These injuries can lead to a series of mini traumas that, in some instances, cause the microglia to be chronically activated. This can create a state of inflammation in the brain.[15, 16]

When there is inflammation, there is interference in the way neurons and neurotransmitters do their jobs, and what you will see is what we see in the classroom—children who are suddenly unable to carry out tasks that they once could with minimal challenge, or changes in personality and students not seeming like themselves. Parents usually notice these changes, too, but they may not know what to do. We would advise parents to seek out a doctor or center that specializes in brain injury. Integrative medical doctors can take a deeper look at something like brain inflammation and suggest a course of treatment. Additionally, specific therapies, such as neurofeedback, have shown promising results for children who have had multiple head traumas. There will be more on those therapies in chapter 10.

We hope that you have come away from this chapter understanding that there are at least some "predictable" aspects of babies growing into toddlers, then into young children, and finally into young adults. Having knowledge of this information can guide you in your ability to parent effectively. It can also arm you with information to discuss with pediatricians and educators if you are concerned about your child's progress. Sometimes, despite our greatest efforts, our children struggle, and this is where we encourage you to reach out to professionals who can help navigate through those temporary roadblocks.

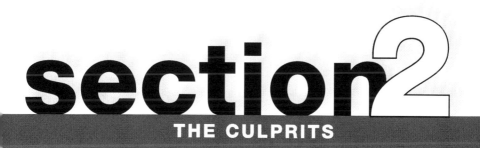

section2

THE CULPRITS

Chapter four

Food and Nutrition: What You Need to Know

"The kinds of food we eat have a direct, chemical based effect on us from the first bite we take in the morning to the last snack before bedtime. Food modifies our hormones. It can improve or impair our metabolism. It can increase or decrease our energy levels. It can strengthen or weaken our concentration and brain performance."

—Natalie Geary, MD, and Oz Garcia, PhD

"My tummy hurts," complains Katie. "I'm hungry," says Michael. Stevie lays his head down on the desk and says he's tired. It's only 9:30 a.m. David rushes into the classroom because "we just got up." Upon being asked if he had taken the time to have breakfast, his response was that he "had the blue juice." The blue dye present on his lips validates his statement. "I had some crackers," chimes in one student. "We didn't have anything in the refrigerator, so I had a pop tart," says another. Then the chorus chimes in, "We didn't have time for breakfast because we were in a hurry," "I didn't eat breakfast because I wasn't hungry," or "I had Captain Crunch."

Answers like these point to a growing trend of minimally nutritious breakfasts with limited or no protein, "nonfood" items, or nothing at all. By the time children arrive at school, many have been up since 7 a.m. or earlier. Because most kids eat their breakfast shortly after rising, that breakfast will have been eaten one to two hours prior to arrival at school. Therefore, unless they have consumed a breakfast rich in protein and healthy fat, chances are their blood sugar is crashing and by 10:00 a.m., they are in a slump and not at all prepared to do schoolwork for another hour or two before lunchtime.

After lunch or snack time, we are met with different kinds of challenges. It is not unusual to see kids return from lunch with stains from the artificial dyes of ice pops on the skin around their lips. If you are on cafeteria duty and you patrol the aisles, you will see a lot of prepackaged foods, such as bags of cookies and cakes, artificial fruit rollups, and candy bars. For some children, if their lunch or snack lacks protein or other nutrient-dense food, we will see mood swings, hyperactivity, or a struggle to stay focused; this hinders their ability to focus and learn in the classroom for the rest of the day.

Well aware of the press coverage on the negatives of processed foods, we decided to dig more deeply into the subject of food. We started thinking carefully about what kind of impact food has on the developing brains and bodies of young children and their behavior and performance in the classroom. Our research led us to focus on two key questions: (1) Are there problematic ingredients in the food supply that could be impacting children and their behavior and ability to learn? (2) Are there specific nutrients a child needs to function optimally? One thing quickly became clear: food has changed. Most foods in the modern diet barely satisfy our genetic requirements. In the words of Drs. Geary and Garcia, experts in children's nutrition, today's food "does not fulfill food's primary functions of providing the mortar for building healthy bodies and brains and the nutrients we need to live longer and well."[1]

Before fast and packaged foods were available, parents had no choice but to purchase whole foods. The advent of packaged foods with a shelf life brought about convenience. We do understand that some foods can be easier to deal with when packing school lunches or for days spent at the ball field, especially when there is concern about food spoilage, but prepackaged, highly preserved foods bring about a host of health and potential behavior problems.

Some doctors have recognized a link between the modern diet and many medical conditions, such as chronic ear infections, bronchitis, acid reflux, skin rashes, low energy, poor or excessive weight gain, and moodiness. Drs. Geary and Garcia connect many of the aforementioned conditions to food intolerance, a topic rarely addressed in mainstream medicine. These are not life-threatening food reactions but can be life-altering reactions nonetheless. Did you know that an intolerance to milk or wheat can lead to chronic ear infections? Or that an intolerance to gluten can cause stomach aches, gas, bloating, constipation, or even irritable bowel syndrome (IBS)?[2] Continuing to eat foods that your body is intolerant to causes inflammation in the gut and eventually the brain.

I want to take a moment to talk about food intolerances. As everyone reading our book now well knows, my older daughter was very ill as a baby and spent the first few years of her life dealing with acid reflux, poor growth, and eczema. Before we had gotten to the integrative medical doctor whom she now sees, she had been tested for immunoglobulin E (IgE) food allergies. IgE food allergies are serious, as they can cause hives or swelling, as well as life-threatening anaphylaxis. When doctors suspect IgE allergies, they typically send you to an allergist for skin prick testing. Or, unfortunately, sometimes IgE allergies are discovered when a child has a life-threatening reaction to a food. We were told our daughter was only IgE allergic to three foods. This didn't make much sense to me, because I could consistently see skin reactions develop following the ingestion of certain foods. Our new doctor introduced me to the concept of food intolerances, otherwise known as immunoglobulin G (IgG) food allergies. IgG food allergies can cause symptoms such as headaches, rashes, and reflux, to name just a few. She tested my daughter for 200+ of the most common foods and seasonings, and as it turned out she was intolerant to well over 100 of them. Of course, we were devastated by these results, but then our doctor explained that what we needed to do was avoid these foods for a period of time while we focused on strengthening her gut and digestive system. Once her gut health was restored, she would be able to eat a more varied diet. Well, let me say that as soon as we eliminated those foods, the eczema that covered her from head to toe, which was not overly responsive to topical steroids, began to clear, and it cleared without any steroids at all. All of her symptoms began to improve when we eliminated the IgG food offenders. Her traditional allergist scoffed at this and told me that he didn't feel IgG food allergies were a "big deal." But our results said otherwise. After healing my daughter's gut, she is now able to eat almost all the foods she once had to avoid. If you suspect your child has symptoms related to a particular food(s), I encourage you to eliminate that food and then see if there is improvement. Eliminating one food at a time, and doing so for three weeks or longer, which is how long it takes to clear out old food proteins and to notice a difference, or work with a doctor who will run IgG food allergy testing.

—Monica

Science is showing us that when you consistently eat a food that you are intolerant to, it causes inflammation in the gut, and that the inflammatory cells involved make their way to the brain.[3,4,5] There is a growing body of evidence that inflammation in the brain prevents the process of synaptic pruning. (We discussed the importance of synaptic pruning in the brain and child development chapters.) One of the most fascinating explanations we have seen on the impact of brain inflammation in the developing child comes from Dr. Patrick Nemechek who says that when synaptic pruning is slowed by inflammation, developmental delays may result.[6] This is because inflammation slows down neuronal communication, leading to delayed rather than quick communication within the brain and body. This makes a lot of sense considering the number of children being diagnosed with food allergies, as well as the number of children being diagnosed with developmental delays. Do the two have to go hand in hand? No. But if your child is experiencing developmental delays, you may want to see a doctor who can help you rule out underlying food intolerances as a cause.

Dr. Sears, a well-known and highly regarded pediatrician, has actually come up with a label for the behavior he is seeing in young children who are frequently misdiagnosed as having ADHD, and that is "Nutritional Deficit Disorder." He describes these children as being hyperactive, irritable, difficult, sleep disordered, and learning or behaving poorly at school and cites the lack of nutrient-dense foods as the culprit.[7]

We want to be clear that we are not saying that ADD is simply a result of poor or inadequate nutrition. We know from brain studies that ADD/ADHD is a real neurological disorder, and there is a visible difference in the brains of children with ADD/ADHD. However, many of the diagnosed cases that are not substantiated by educational testing or brain studies may actually be cleared up by reevaluating and making changes to your child's diet.

We see children in the classroom every day who appear to be suffering from what we believe are food-related issues that have real consequences on behavior and learning. We hope that this chapter will help parents realize that a connection between food, behavior, and learning may not be picked up on in a quick visit to the doctor, and that deeper investigation may be warranted.

The Quiet Culprits in Our Food Supply

While there are many issues of concern surrounding our food supply, we have chosen to highlight some of the ones we feel parents should be most aware of.

Dyes and Preservatives

A growing body of evidence links food dyes and preservatives to hyperactive behavior. So significant were the findings of multiple studies that the European Union has banned certain food additives and now requires the following label be placed on food packages that contain any one of six artificial dyes or preservatives that have fallen under scrutiny: "may have an adverse effect on activity and attention in children." The U.S. government has often been criticized for being slow to respond to concerns about the food supply. Dr. Joel Nigg, professor of psychiatry, pediatrics and behavioral neuroscience at Oregon Health & Science University, says, "Do you want to take a chance that these initial studies are wrong and put kids at risk or do you want to take a chance that they're right? We have to work on the data we have."[8] Pediatrician Dr. Benjamin Feingold has been trying to raise the red flag about dyes and preservatives in America since the 1970s and is the founder of an elimination diet plan that has helped to dramatically improve behavioral problems in many children.[9]

Added Sweeteners

Aspartame

This is a highly controversial ingredient, which many senior officials at the Food and Drug Administration (FDA) voted against approving because of the high rate of brain tumors found in animals that were exposed to it. There also have been no long-term human studies of this additive. In humans, symptoms related to aspartame ingestion can be hypoglycemia (a condition involving the body's regulation of blood sugar), headaches, dizziness, depression, anxiety, sleep disturbance, and a host of other symptoms. Aspartame is a sweet substance—200 times sweeter than real cane sugar—and therefore it can be used in small quantities, which reduces the calorie amounts in food. Aspartame is used in most diet sodas and many other sweetened drinks, as well as in many commercial candy and gum products. Take a look at the tiny print list of ingredients on your favorite gums or candies, and you will likely find it listed as an ingredient.[10,11]

Following a 2014 survey that showed the 5.2 percent dip in sales due to consumer concern over aspartame, Pepsi Corporation announced it was pulling it from Diet Pepsi. A long-term study done by Columbia University showed that drinking just one diet soda with aspartame as the sweetener a day led to a 43 percent increase in risk of heart attack and stroke. A similar study done at the University of Minnesota showed the risk of diabetes is raised by 36 percent for those who drink one diet soda a day. A study done at the University of Texas Health Science Center in San Antonio showed that those who drink one diet soda a day have a 41 percent increased risk of obesity. Given the rise of obesity and diabetes in American children, it seems like aspartame and diet soda are well worth avoiding.[12]

Defenders of aspartame will tell you not to worry about the potential side effects; they argue that the animal studies exposed the animals to super high doses of aspartame, amounts much greater than a human would consume in a serving. While it may be true that these animals were exposed to more than humans would consume in a single serving, when you consider the amount of servings of aspartame you consume across all food products you eat each day, it is easy to see how very quickly you may be entering into super high-dose territory.

Corn Syrup and High Fructose Corn Syrup

Although these are technically two different compounds, both cause similar concerns. Corn syrup was developed in the 1950s but wasn't added widely into the food supply until the 1970s. Corn syrup was developed as a money-saver for large food corporations. Like aspartame, you can use less of this sweetening agent than real sugar while achieving a "sweeter" effect. In his book, *The End of Overeating: Taking Control of the Insatiable American Appetite*, David Kessler, the former head of the FDA, writes about the evidence he claims he saw during his tenure there, that corn syrup and substitute sugars are as addictive as cigarettes or alcohol.[13] A study conducted by the Princeton Neuroscience Institute in 2010 showed that rats, once introduced to corn syrup in their food supply, actively sought it out (i.e., craved it), and when it was taken away from them the rats displayed withdrawal behaviors, similar to those of humans withdrawing from drugs or alcohol.[14]

This offers a plausible explanation for why our children crave and actively seek out processed foods containing corn syrup and high fructose corn syrup once they have been introduced into their diet (and why they may become very unhappy with us when we try to take those foods away). Studies have shown that as these artificial sweeteners exit our bodies, people experience withdrawal-like symptoms, such as nervousness, anxiousness, and the jitters, causing the person to want to experience relief—and what causes relief? Getting more of the substance back into the body! So again, it is no wonder to us that people crave these foods and that so many people, children in particular, have become overweight as a byproduct.

Chemicals

Many foods are packaged in plastic or cans. In the 1960s a new chemical called bisphenol-A (BPA) was added into plastic products. BPA was used to line baby bottles, bottles of drinking water, canned infant formulas, and to this day it is still in the lining of many plastic and metal canned goods (including many brands of bottled water). It has been proven that in certain quantities BPA is neurotoxic, meaning, a substance that is poisonous or destructive to nerves and nerve tissue. While a single exposure to something like BPA may not cause an issue, if one were constantly bombarded with exposures via the use of everyday products, there could be a buildup of that chemical in the body. In 2010, the FDA finally banned the use of BPA in infant products,[15] and many manufacturers have voluntarily taken this chemical out of their water bottles and plastic products. However, it is still in many common household products. For example, BPA is in the liner of a host of canned food products. Many brands have begun to clearly share on their labels that their packaging is BPA-free.

So why should you be concerned? Measurable amounts of BPA have been found in the urine, breast milk, and umbilical cords of newborn babies. In August 2008, the National Toxicology Program of the National Institute of Environmental Health Services showed that exposure to BPA can cause undesirable neural and behavioral effects in fetuses, infants. and children.[16] A Yale University study had similar findings.[17]

In a 2004 study funded by the Environmental Working Group, the umbilical cords of newborn babies were tested for the presence of some 400 chemicals. Their study found 287 of those chemicals to be present in the umbilical cords of those babies; 180 of those chemicals are known to cause cancer in humans and animals, and

217 are known to be toxic to the brain and nervous system. A 2009 follow-up study by the same group found equally disturbing results.[18]

A very unfortunate accident helped scientists learn that the developing brain of fetuses, infants and young children are far more susceptible to being injured by chemicals and metals in the environment than a mature brain. In the 1950s, a toxic mercury spill from an industrial plant got into the water supply serving Minamata, Japan. Autopsies on the adults who suffered from mercury toxicity showed that there were lesions caused by the mercury in some parts of the brain; however, in the fetuses of the pregnant adult women who died from toxic exposure neuronal death and damage to the nervous system was greater than that in the adults.[19] Scientists at the University of Minnesota offer a deeper discussion on the subject of mercury, sharing that mercury does tend to make its way to the brain and is a neurotoxin. They also highlight a study carried out in New Zealand, which revealed poorer scores on full-scale IQ, language development, visual-spatial skills, and gross motor skills in the children of mothers who had a higher level of mercury found in their hair.[20]

So how did these chemicals get into our food and environment? As of the printing of this book, there are over 75,000 synthetic chemicals in use. In the 1960s and 1970s, the development of chemicals and synthetic products became a booming industry in the United States. In 1976, the Toxic Substance Control Act was approved. While at a quick glance, this sounds like an act that might have been designed to protect people, it seems just the opposite occurred. This act requires the government to approve or deny a new chemical proposed for approval within 90 days. If you read the act itself, you'll learn that very little testing is required of the companies seeking approval of their chemical, and it is actually the government's responsibility to prove that the chemical is unsafe![21] Something seems terribly wrong that so little testing is done before chemicals make their way into our environment and into products we come into contact with. If you are anything like us, right now you are feeling a little upset that our children have essentially been treated like guinea pigs or test subjects.

The good news is that on June 22, 2016, the Frank R. Lautenberg Chemical Safety for the 21st Century Act was signed into law, amending the Toxic Substances Control Act (TSCA). This law has stricter testing requirements and guidelines, which is a start to offering better protection from potentially harmful chemicals.[22]

What Do We Really Know About GMOs?

A genetically modified food is one where there have been changes introduced into the DNA of the food via genetic engineering. Genetically modified foods can be a whole food, such as a type of potato or a type of apple. A GMO can also be in a food product, such as cereal which may contain multiple food ingredients, some of which may be genetically modified. One purpose of GMOs is to make them resistant to pests, allowing farmers to grow more food. Sounds great in theory, but in actuality there are many issues with this. Journalist Michael Pollan has raised many concerning issues about GMOs after extensively researching the topic for the *New York Times*. Focusing on a breed of GMO potatoes that contain an insecticide called New Leaf, he questioned how the presence of the insecticide may affect consumers and how the potato would be labeled for sale. When he posed these questions to Monsanto, the agrochemical and agricultural biotechnology giant that created New Leaf potatoes, he was told that because a pesticide is not a food, it does not require labeling by the FDA. However, if the insecticide was sold on the shelf of home improvement stores, the EPA would require labeling about its safety. Because the EPA does not have jurisdiction over food products, it cannot require labeling in that context.

When Pollan asked Philip Angell, Monsanto's director of communications, whether he was concerned about the safety of the New Leaf potato, he replied, "Monsanto should not have to vouch for the safety of biotech food. Our interest is in selling as much of it is possible. Assuring its safety is the FDA's job." Pollan then researched the FDA's position on the matter and found the following statement in FDA (GMO Policy) Federal Register Vol. 57, Number 104 (1992), page 229: "Ultimately it is the food producer who is responsible for assuring safety."

As parents and educators, it is a very frightening to us that that there appears to be no checks and balances in place to regulate the safety of GMO foods. Meanwhile it continues to be a thriving industry, with over 45 million acres of farmland in America being used to grow GMO crops. Some of the most commonly consumed foods in the American diet (soy, corn, and potato) are being sold on the shelves of supermarkets, GMO label free.[23]

Another purpose of GMO foods is to give the food the ability to withstand massive spraying of Round Up. The main ingredient in the commercial product Round Up is glyphosate. This is a chemical herbicide used by many private citizens to kill weeds on their lawn and by commercial agriculture to kill threats to their crops. The idea is to "protect" farming, allowing the greatest yield of the crops to get to the supermarket shelf. Again, it sounds great in theory; however, the human body only has systems to recognize the foods that are natural to this Earth. We are changing the nature of our food and potentially causing a problem for the human body to recognize it. Maybe more important, if Round Up is sprayed on many commercial foods and you are eating most of these commercially grown foods, over time your body is ingesting large quantities of glyphosate. Now, the scientists and large corporations behind the concept of GMOs have a quick and handy answer for folks as to why this isn't a problem: they will tell you that Round Up doesn't affect humans. They will say that it acts on something called the "shikimate pathway," which plant-based crops possess but that humans do not. However, they will leave out a very important piece of information: the good bacteria, which all humans possess in the gut and need for the proper breakdown and digestion of food, does contain this pathway. Therefore, the Round Up is affecting our good gut bacteria and throws off our digestive process. This seems to be a problem we should be concerned about. Not only are we ingesting glyphosate via some of the foods we are eating, but also commercial animals are often fed GMO corn, soy, and vegetable diets. Therefore, the nonorganic meat most are buying also contains glyphosate.[24]

A study printed in the journal *Environmental and Analytical Toxicology* found that glyphosate accumulated in the bodies of all the animals tested. In particular, it accumulated in the bones, interfered with the synthesis of critical neurotransmitters, and led to nutrient deficiencies. The researchers also found glyphosate in higher concentration in the urine of chronically ill humans as compared to humans who were not ill.[25] Glyphosate has been banned in many major European nations. Glyphosate has been found in high quantities in the breast milk of American women, at anywhere from 760 to 1,600 times the allowable limits in European drinking water, and urine tests of Americans have shown 10 times the glyphosate accumulation as Europeans.[26] MIT researcher Dr. Stephanie Seneff has been studying glyphosate for several decades, and has over 170 peer-reviewed scholarly articles. She claims there is a direct relationship between glyphosate and many health-related conditions such as autism, Alzheimer's disease, and cardiovascular disease. A study done in the state of California showed a 60 percent increase in the risk of autism of children born to mothers living near farms where glyphosate-based pesticides are used in great quantity.[27,28]

Unfortunately, the DARK Bill of 2016 was passed and signed into law. This bill makes it so that food manufacturers are not legally required to share with consumers whether the food they are eating is a genetically modified food or not. This creates more work for you; we encourage you to research the food you buy and look for the organic or GMO-free label wherever and whenever you can!

If you are worried about your family's exposure to toxins, there is some good news. Science has shown that chemicals actually exit the body relatively quickly. A study conducted by the Swedish Environmental Research Institute in conjunction with the Coop supermarket chain tracked pesticides entering and exiting the human body. The group provided a family with completely organic food for two weeks. Prior to eating the organic food, the family had been eating nonorganic foods available in most supermarkets. Urine samples were taken from the mother, father, and three children. Measurable amounts of insecticide, fungicide, plant growth regulators, and 12 common pesticides were found in all urine samples. After eating strictly organic for two weeks, urine samples were again taken, and levels of the pesticides had dropped to trace amounts or were gone altogether.[29] A similar study in Australia on 26 adults showed that after eating a mainly organic diet for just one week, over 89 percent of the toxins initially found in the urine were gone![30] Obviously eating organic as much as possible is one great way to avoid toxins; however, there are two other inexpensive ways to rid the body of toxins. Sweating it out through exercise is one great way to eliminate toxins from the body, and exercise carries many other health benefits.[31] Also, drinking plenty of clean filtered water daily helps your kidneys and liver flush toxins from your system.[32] We tend to forget that water itself is an essential nutrient. Water transports nutrients and oxygen to our cells, it helps maintain blood volume, and helps lubricate joints. Children should be drinking five to eight cups of water a day.[33]

While we may not be able to fully control the bad things our children are exposed to, with knowledge of proper nutrition and the role of vitamins and minerals, we can take steps to build our children up. Entire books have been written on nutrition, and our book is not one of them, but we do want to outline recommended nutrient intake for children and offer some tips and tricks that you can use to improve your family's diet.

What Nutrients Do Kids Need?

Ages 5 to 14

Girls—range from 1200–2000 calories	
FOOD CATEGORY	SERVING SIZE
Protein:	3-6 ounces
Fruit:	1-2 cups
Vegetables:	1.5-3 cups
Grains:	4-7 ounces
Dairy:	2.5-3 cups

Boys—range from 1400–2600 calories	
FOOD CATEGORY	SERVING SIZE
Protein:	3-6.5 ounces
Fruit:	1-2 cups
Vegetables:	1.5-3.5 cups
Grains:	4-9 ounces
Dairy:	2.5-3 cups

These numbers aren't arbitrary; they are based on what the body requires to be able to function properly. Please be aware that these are broad figures, and that some children have differing nutritional needs. If you are concerned as to whether your child is getting proper nutrition through dietary choices, consult a doctor or nutritionist. We know that getting kids to consume a healthy diet is not always easy, which is why we have included tips and strategies to help implement a healthier approach to food in your households at the end of the chapter.

Have you ever experienced feeling really hungry shortly after you just ate a bunch of "stuff?" Or do you ever find yourself "foraging" in the kitchen pantry or refrigerator, not knowing exactly what you want, but you know you want something to eat? The human body seeks the nutrients it needs from the food that has gone into the digestive system. Because those nutrients are not found in processed foods, the body continues to search for what it needs. It sends the brain signals to eat more, hoping that in the next round of food it will get the nutrients it needs. Most are surprised to find that when they change their diet to whole nutrient-dense foods, their appetite and resultant overeating decreases, and thus weight loss, more energy, and fewer cravings follow.

Macronutrients

Protein

Protein is a component of every cell in the body and is an important building block for bones, cartilage, muscles, skin, and blood. Our bodies use protein to build and repair tissues and to make enzymes, hormones, and other chemicals used by the body. Unlike fats and carbohydrates, the body cannot store protein, which is why it needs to be consumed more frequently.[34] Healthy sources of protein include organic grass-fed beef, seafood, chicken, pork, eggs, beans, and dairy products like cheese and yogurt.[35]

Carbohydrates

Carbohydrates are the fiber, sugars, and starches found in vegetables, fruits, and grains and can be broken down into two groups: simple or complex. They are one of the body's primary sources of energy, and they play an important role in the central nervous system and brain function.[36] Simple carbohydrates are digested quickly and rapidly elevate blood sugar. Examples include fruit, fruit juices, and honey.[37] Complex carbohydrates, in contrast, take longer for the body to break down and lead to more sustained periods of energy.[38] Examples are whole grains, starchy vegetables, and beans.[39]

Fat

An underappreciated macronutrient, fat, has earned the reputation as the "bad guy," and unfortunately this is only partially true. The good kind of fat is the kind that is less saturated, examples being omega-3 and omega-6. Good fat helps fuel the body, providing energy and creating healthy cell membranes. Good fat helps build something called myelin, a cushion that surrounds our nerves. Remember we previously discussed how there is a massive network of nerves and neurons throughout the body. When nerves are surrounded by a healthy layer of myelin, they communicate much more quickly. Eating good fats helps build a smarter brain. Fat also helps the body absorb important vitamins such as A, D, E and K, all of which are essential to developing healthy eyes![40] Perhaps most important, fat helps the body feel full.[41] A breakfast consisting of a whole egg (not just an egg white) and whole cheese, not reduced-fat cheese, will hold the body hours longer because it takes the body longer to break down and digest the fat. Good fats also do something very important; they help carry bad cholesterol (LDL) out of the body. Fat also gives food flavor. Did you ever notice how delicious a good steak that has a healthy layer of fat on it tastes? When food manufacturers created low- and nonfat foods, they realized quickly they lacked flavor and substituted in lots of sugar to compensate.[42]

Fat can be bad, especially excessive amounts of the highly saturated kind: hydrogenated, partially hydrogenated, and trans fats. However, some good quality butter or whole milk cream cheese spread on a bagel or toast is okay. Just remember moderation is the key.

Like fat, cholesterol has had a bad reputation for many decades. During the Framingham Study conducted in 1948, scientists and doctors discovered that fat and cholesterol were what was inside the bad plaque found inside human hearts following a heart attack. As a result of the findings of this study, the medical field suggested a low-fat and low-cholesterol diet. Unfortunately, at the time of the Framingham Study, the equipment wasn't sophisticated enough to see the whole picture and led to the premature conclusion that all fat and cholesterol were bad. Newer advances in science have shown that the dietary recommendations made as a result of this study were wrong. The human body requires a certain amount of fat and cholesterol to function properly. Cholesterol helps the body produce vitamin D; it helps with cellular repair and with the proper function of many hormones. Eighty percent of the body's supply of cholesterol is made within the body itself, but when you don't have enough cholesterol in your body, your body reacts by producing more of it, creating a much bigger problem. There are two kinds of cholesterol, and we need more of the good kind (HDL) and less of the bad kind (LDL). Remember that healthy fats help carry bad cholesterol out of the bloodstream.

Healthy sources of fat include avocados, whole milk cheese, tree nuts (and nut butters), seeds, fish, olives (olive oil), and, believe it or not, dark chocolate![43]

One consequence of eating food that is not nutrient dense can be vitamin deficiencies. The following are some examples of what these deficiencies can look like (you might recognize how these could impact learning).

Micronutrients and Deficiencies

Vitamin D deficiency can lead to frequent illness (i.e., colds, viruses, and bacterial infections), a sweaty head, weak muscles, and/or fatigue, feeling sad/blue with no identifiable cause, weak/soft bones and teeth (leading to frequent breaks or cavities), and asthma.[44]

The CDC reports that 32 percent of children are vitamin D deficient—that's approximately one in every three children! Because many are unable to get enough vitamin D from natural exposure to sunlight, a vitamin D supplement might be necessary.[45]

Magnesium deficiency can lead to muscle weakness, muscle cramps, constipation, difficulty sleeping, nausea, anxiety, and poor memory.[46]

Iron deficiency can lead to loss of appetite, fatigue, irritability, pale skin, irregular heartbeat, and dizziness.[47]

The B vitamins include B_1 (thiamine), B_2 (riboflavin), B_3 (niacinamide), B_5 (pantothenic acid), B_6 (pyridoxine), B_9 (folic acid), and B_{12} (cobalamin). They are the backbone of many bodily functions, including energy production, metabolic function, circulation, synthesis and breakdown of amino acids, digestion of fat and carbohydrates, and DNA and RNA synthesis—just to name a few![48] The following are symptoms of specific B vitamin deficiencies:[49]

- B_1—depression, constipation, weakness, irritability, loss of appetite, loss of weight, insomnia
- B_2—sluggishness, itching and burning eyes, cracked lips or sores in the mouth or on lips, digestive disturbance, trembling, oily skin
- B_3—depression, nervousness, insomnia, headaches, skin disorders, poor growth, canker sores, pellagra
- B_5—restlessness, painful and burning feet, slow growth, dizzy spells, vomiting, muscle cramping
- B_6—insomnia, skin eruptions, loss of muscle control, anemia, loss of hair, delayed learning, water retention
- B_9—gastrointestinal disorders, anemia, B12 deficiency, premature graying of hair
- B_{12}—depression, fatigue, pernicious anemia, poor appetite, poor growth, poor balance

Zinc deficiency can lead to diarrhea, poor growth, a weakened immune system, poor wound healing, poor learning and memory, and even fertility problems.[50] Zinc deficiency can lead to a loss of taste and smell, which, in turn, can lead to a poor appetite, picky eating and potentially weight loss.[51] Zinc is an essential trace element that is involved in stimulating the activity of over 100 enzymes in the body. It is considered the backbone of the immune system because it helps regulate proper immune responses and aids in the attack of infected or cancerous cells. Zinc is involved in wound healing, in preventing or controlling diarrhea, and in regulating how neurons communicate with one another (remember, we talked about the importance of neuron function in the brain chapter).

If you are concerned that your child may have nutrient deficiencies, you could talk with his or her doctor about ordering some diagnostic bloodwork.

Tips and Tricks to Make Healthy Changes

Eating a diet grounded in whole, nutrient-dense foods provides the body with the fuel it needs to run optimally. We understand that getting young children to eat healthy is not always easy. So here are some tips that we've tested in our own kitchens, with our children, and with our local clients! In chapter 9, we offer additional ideas and strategies for healthy eating.

> *I consider myself to be a pretty well-informed parent and a healthy eater. Despite this, I have faced my own significant challenges in getting each of my children to eat certain foods. I think it is important to emphasize here that there is no one size fits all model. When you look at different nutrient groups, don't feel like you have to have your children eating a broad variety within each group. While that would be nice, the reality is that if they have only one or two favorites within each group, this is better than none. Don't feel bad if you have to use some of the "sneaky" tips—it doesn't matter how the food gets in*

there—just get it in! You don't want to have food become a huge source of stress. Instead set the intention to start making positive and healthy changes and recognize that for some kids and households it is going to take longer than others! Remember to have patience with yourself and your children!

—Monica

Tip 1: A diet is not punishment. Many well-meaning parents say things like, "The doctor said you are overweight so I am throwing out all the 'garbage' in our pantry and we are starting a diet tomorrow," or "We've decided that we are eating really unhealthy food, so tomorrow we start healthy food boot camp." Instead, say something like, "As a family, we want to start making healthier choices. By eating the right foods, we can have more energy and do better at our jobs, school and on the athletic field." Then start teaching children about making choices that include protein and healthy fat, and let them know why too many carbohydrates can be a problem. Start filling your pantry and fridge with better options that children can reach and moving the foods that you are trying to remove to a higher place where they can't access it without asking you first.

Tip 2: Set realistic expectations. Drs. Geary and Garcia mention that research shows it can take 8 to 10 tries of something new to acquire the taste for it![52] Negotiate with your children that all you require of them is to try one forkful or one spoonful of the new item. Do that for 8 to 10 days. Then increase that to two forkfuls, and then a week later to three. As you increase the amount of good food going in, your children should notice a difference in how they feel, and will likely, over time, not only eat the new choice but also understand it makes them feel better! We all have taste buds that acquire a taste, but taste buds can and do change!

Tip 3: Talk to your kids about food. You might think this sounds silly, but it works. When you get out food, tell your child what it is, and why it is important to eat it. For example, explain why protein is good. "This bowl of chili will give you more energy. These apple slices have natural sugar that will give you energy and fiber which will help you feel full so that you don't run out of steam during the game." The more you do this, kids start to ask questions about food, like, "Mom is this good for me?" Kids start to take pride in their food choices and may say something like, "Dad, aren't you proud of me, I chose a healthy snack." Be sure to reinforce them for making wise choices. Parents tend to underestimate the impact of their positive feedback.

Tip 4: Fool the veggie haters. Here's a strategy to try for vegetable "haters." Look in the refrigerator section of your grocery store for juice smoothies. The brand Bolthouse Farms makes a drink called "Green Goodness." Now, it is green, so you've got to get creative. Find a cup that is a solid color (i.e., not see through). If they see green, they are probably going to refuse. Then say to your child, "Hey, take a quick sip of this new drink I found." You might even use a solid color straw so that they don't catch site of the green at all. This drink provides spirulina, broccoli, spinach, Jerusalem artichoke, and a host of other great things, including apple, pineapple, mango, banana, and kiwi (so now you've got some of your fruit intake covered, too). This drink is gluten and dairy free and free of preservatives and artificial colors and flavors. Yes, it contains sugar (no added sugar), but it is natural sugar from the fruit that the human body recognizes and needs a certain amount of! While one container of Green Goodness can be pricey, most supermarkets run sales and wholesale food clubs often carry this exact drink offering 64 ounces for the same price as the 15.2-ounce version at the supermarket! There are other versions, so keep trying until you find the right one. Even if you find a smoothie that contains ONE vegetable, this may be one more vegetable than your child ate yesterday.

Another trick for the picky vegetable eater is to steam or sauté the vegetables with sea salt. There is a HUGE difference between sea salt and table salt. Table salt not only has no nutritional value, it is loaded with sodium and can drive up blood pressure. Pink sea salt, on the other hand, is loaded with micronutrients. You can heap on the sea salt and only add value to the meal, and for many kids that extra flavor of the sea salt makes vegetable more palatable.[53] Cooking vegetables in organic butter, ghee, or coconut oil are other ways to add flavor that might make them more palatable to those who have an aversion to the taste of vegetables.

Tip 5: Use healthy seasonings. Some seasonings that make meat and vegetables taste better are olive oil, sea salt, and a good quality butter. Most kids like salty things, so again, in an effort to convert them, don't be afraid to use these seasonings to make different foods more palatable! Small amounts can pack a lot of flavor, and these are readily available in supermarkets! Olive oil and butter add a dose of omega—3 fatty acids, and sea salt contributes many essential micronutrients!

Tip 6: Pack a punch at breakfast. Few cereals contain protein or healthy fats, and the ones that do often do not contain enough to make a difference. We understand morning time can be chaotic, and cereal is fast and easy. But if you can carve just 15 extra minutes into your morning routine, you can likely shift from cereal to other options. Because children are creatures of habit, don't upset their apple cart. As you keep that cereal on board, slowly try adding in one of the following as a "side dish."

- *Eggs*—If you can make an omelet with veggies even better, two forkfuls of eggs in addition to the usual cereal is better than none; consider making mini omelets in a cupcake pan for on-the-run breakfasts or snacks.

- *Bacon*—A good quality one, perhaps uncured, will offer protein and healthy fat.

- *Plain whole Greek yogurt*—Add a little honey and fresh berries and/or nuts; again two spoonfuls of this concoction in addition to the usual breakfast is better than nothing.

- *Apple slices with a nut butter*—If tree nuts or peanuts are a problem, Sun Butter is a great solution. In fact, it contains just four simple ingredients and has 7 grams of protein and 16 grams of healthy fat (brain fuel) per serving.

Tip 7: Make simple swaps. Mix a small amount of the new thing into whatever they normally eat. For example, start with their regular peanut butter and add a teaspoon of Sun Butter into it. Over time, back out the peanut butter and up the Sun Butter. If peanuts aren't a problem, try converting from a peanut butter that has lots of sugar and corn syrup to an organic one made with a healthy oil. You can do this trick with yogurt as well. It was shocking to discover that the average single-serving Greek yogurt container has 18 to 24 grams of sugar! Kids are used to that sweet taste, so put the yogurt in a plastic storage container and slowly start adding one tablespoon of plain whole fat Greek yogurt into the original one they have been eating and stir well. Over time as their taste buds start losing the taste for that super sweetness, you can add in more and more tablespoons of the plain whole version. You can also do this with iced teas and other juices by slowly adding in a healthier unsweetened version.

Tip 8: Add omega fatty acids and fish:

- Use olive oil judiciously when cooking, and a good quality, organic brand if possible!

- Sneak in something like avocado by whipping even just a small amount into your mashed potatoes.

- Use good quality nut butters as spreads on apple slices, in sandwiches, or on toast.

- Cook or grill fish with fresh squeezed lemon to take away the "fishy" taste or at least minimize it. But then also add on melted butter or try some breading. Also, you may want to start with a fish that is less fishy overall, like flounder; a fried piece of buttered and breaded flounder might almost pass as a chicken tender!

- For kids who just will not try a bite of fish, consider a high-quality supplement such as Nordic Naturals Omega 3 Gummy Fish (if the sight of fish is a problem, they make a sour gummy worm). Of course, if you use gummy supplements, your dentist will tell you to be sure your children are brushing their teeth well, as some of the sticky pieces can get lodged in the crevices of the teeth, leading to an increase in cavities.

Tip 9: Drink clean water. Many products are on the market that allow parents to access cleaner water than what comes out of the tap, such as filter based jugs, filters that attach to faucets, and whole-house filtration systems that can be installed to clean out all water coming into the home from the public water pipeline.

Tip 10: Reduce toxins on a budget:

Clean Fifteen™

The "Clean 15" are the fruits and veggies that are the most free of pesticides, so it is not as important to buy organic:[54]

- Avocados

- Sweet corn

- Pineapple

- Cabbage

- Frozen sweet peas

- Onions

- Asparagus

- Mangoes

- Papayas

- Kiwis

- Eggplant

- Cantaloupe

- Grapefruit

- Cauliflower

- Sweet potatoes

Dirty Dozen™

The "Dirty Dozen" are fruits and veggies that are sprayed most heavily with pesticides, so it's best to buy organic if you can:[55]

- Apples

- Strawberries

- Grapes

- Celery

- Peaches

- Spinach

- Sweet bell peppers

- Nectarines

- Cucumbers

- Cherry tomatoes

- Snap peas

- Potatoes

One thing many people don't realize is that frozen organic fruits and vegetables are often cheaper than fresh, so if need be, buy frozen! Another thing to keep in mind is that many major food brands are voluntarily providing labeling to show they are either organic and/or GMO free. Some of those brands are pricier, but we have seen more and more of those brands popping up in large wholesale stores where the pricing is more affordable for many families.

Chapter five

What Happened to Play?

"Play is often talked about as it were a relief from serious learning. But for children, play is serious learning. Play is the work of children."

— Fred Rogers

Every Monday in schools around the country, teachers ask their students, "What did you do this weekend?" Then the students may share the "Weekend News" with their class-mates or write about it in their journals. The tales rarely reflect playing outside due to the weather being too hot or too cold, the family being too busy, or the kids just prefer-ring to stay inside and play the latest video game. Any drive through a suburban neighborhood will look very different today than it did 20 years ago. There may be a few children playing outside or someone walking a child in a stroller. But compared to a generation ago, the garage doors are down, the swings stand still, and very few children race about and play.

These informal observations are supported by the data. The average American child now spends half as much time outside as compared to only 20 years ago.[1] Only 6 percent of children will play outside on their own in a typical week.[2] Dr. Stuart Brown, founding director of the National Institute for Play, says, "Kids are 71 percent less involved in outdoor activities now than they were 10 years ago. To me, it's a public health issue."[3] Overall, Americans now spend 93 percent of their time inside a building or vehicle.[4] Compared to urban and rural kids, suburban kids, those with the most opportunity in some areas, suffer the greatest health and psychological problems from a lack of play. Coupled with the lack of play is an overall lack of interaction with the physical environment in which one lives, the world outside the home or classroom.

In a study that was documented in the film *Where Do the Children Play?* (2008), researchers compared how observant, collaborative, and creative children were when asked to build a pretend neighborhood out of art materials. They were interested in how these traits might differ depending on the environment in which the children were being raised, be it urban, rural, or suburban neighborhoods. What they observed was that suburban children were less observant, less collaborative, and less creative when completing the task compared to urban and rural children. One explanation researchers offered for these results is that children from the suburbs are often chauffeured to events and organized activities. In the car, these children are merely passengers and less observant of their surroundings because it is not required. In many suburban neighborhoods, families arrive home in the car, drive into the garage, and put down the doors. There is less physical interaction with the environment.[5] Furthermore, children who spend a lot of time in cars may be utilizing an in-car video or handheld device, making them even less likely to observe what is going on around them. This is in contrast to the children from urban and rural areas who are "out and about" in their communities. Being outside, in nature or on the street, forces them to be more involved and more aware of their environment.

For centuries, play was just something that naturally happened, but then it didn't. So what happened to play? In our opinion, and that of medical researchers and child development specialists, there are many reasons that play changed, including:

- Advertising on television
- Safety concerns
- Changes in lifestyles and family structure
- Changes in curriculum and high-stakes testing

Advertising

What really changed children's play began in the 1950s with the debut of advertising toys for children on television outside of the Christmas season. According to Howard Chudacoff, a cultural historian at Brown University, children's play became focused on things rather than the action of playing. "It's interesting to me that when we talk about play today, the first thing that comes to mind are toys," says Chudacoff. "Whereas when I would think of play in the 19th century, I would think of activity rather than an object."[6] Toys have changed and don't always nurture creativity and imagination. In addition, as commercialism increased and televisions became more prevalent in our homes, any viewing time was time not spent playing outside.

Safety Concerns

Concerns about safety also changed the environments in which children played. Lessons, leagues, and camps emerged as safe alternatives and ways to enrich the lives of children. However, they do not reap the same benefits as imaginative, free play. We will give camps the benefit of the doubt, because many do offer incredible experiences in nature and nurture many worthwhile, brain-building skills, but for the most part, today's children are more directed, protected, catered to, ranked, judged, and rewarded by adults. It's like everything is being "done to them" rather than "with them."[7] In addition, consider the safety precautions that are in place in today's schools. The level of security and supervision in all arenas is definitely heightened and somewhat limits the spontaneity of children's play. When children no longer have a sense of control, we know their levels of anxiety and depression can increase.[8]

Changes in Lifestyles and Family Structure

Many parents are working long hours, which can result in extra time in daycare or aftercare programs. Some of these programs do not build in a plethora of outdoor or creative playtime. Additionally, there are more extracurricular choices today, and some of them are quite competitive, involve huge time and financial commitments, and can challenge even the most organized, dedicated parent. These activities also are often highly organized, and so while children may seem "at play," it isn't free creative play. Some households have a sense of frenzy about them that impacts the family's ability to relax and spend some time in joyful play or reading bedtime stories.

Changes in School Curriculum

Over the last 20 to 25 years, educational curriculums have been ramped up to reflect new federal- and state-mandated standards and high-stakes testing, with many of these standards being developmentally inappropriate. In order to improve scores on upcoming tests, some students are invited to participate in before or after school tutoring and/or may also qualify for summer school. While it's admirable that some school districts are providing additional support, it does reflect the changes in education and can make for a very long day, which takes time away from family, sleep, relaxation, and play. In addition to an already chock-filled curriculum, many school districts nationwide have found it necessary to create bullying and harassment statements, policies, and protocols, and have adopted and implemented programs that increase awareness about bullying and/or teach social and emotional curriculums across the grade levels.[9,10] Many educators support these programs because, like us, they believe that if students aren't emotionally healthy, it's very difficult to teach academic skills. Remember that when the upstairs brain shuts down, the downstairs brain goes into action, so when students are experiencing mental health issues, they can be in a state of "flight or fight." The feelings of fear, worry, anxiety, panic, or frustration can physically affect the brain's ability to think and remember, which can negate any productive academic learning. However, it can be difficult for educators to fit everything into a school day. The challenge is this: schools are no longer responsible for just academic skill instruction like they were many years ago. Teachers feel pressured to make every minute of instructional time count. There is just too much to do! Can you see why time for free play has decreased?

Even the preschool curriculum tends to reflect society and local school districts' expectations and standards. Because of the emphasis on testing, teachers and well-meaning parents are starting earlier and earlier to drill their kids in the basic fundamentals even if the kids are just not ready. But herein lies the problem that can have long-lasting effects. Preschool years are a critical developmental period. If children are not given enough natural movement and play experiences in a three-dimensional world, they start their academic careers at a disadvantage. Remember the increase in the number of referrals for fine motor problems that we mentioned? Many children are starting formal schooling with underdeveloped hands, resulting in poor handwriting habits that are extremely difficult for a primary educator to change. These habits lead to maladapted grips and illegible, inefficient handwriting.[11] What this translates into are:

- Students who have many good ideas but no efficient means of getting their thoughts down on paper, and therefore their writing isn't commensurate with their cognitive ability

- "Short and sweet" answers because the writing is just too laborious

- Avoidance behaviors during written tasks due to high levels of frustration

- Tired hands and bodies

My own daughter began to feel the pressure of high-stakes tests as early as 4 years old. She perceived that she was not meeting the standards that she was expected to in the classroom and started to become frustrated. For example, she threw down her pencil and said, "Mommy I can't do it." This was very out of character for my even-keeled child who actually takes great pride in doing just about anything herself. I knew something needed to change, so I spoke with her teacher and asked that some of the pressure be taken off the academic part of the program, because to me it felt like too much, too soon. She shared that preschool teachers are being told by kindergarten teachers that the kids need to be more academically "primed" for learning before they arrive to kindergarten, which caused their preschool to "ramp up" the curriculum. This approach was causing my very bright daughter to shut down. Many of my friends are counselors, and they can attest to treating an increasing number of elementary-aged children for school and test anxiety. I also know many educators and administrators who do not agree with pushing a heavy duty academic curriculum down into preschool and kindergarten. Some public schools are trying to work at the state level to reverse what they feel to be inappropriate mandates.

—Monica

Angela Hanscom, pediatric occupational therapist and advocate for play, has also noticed that children are coming to class with bodies that are less prepared to learn than ever before:

> With sensory systems not quite working right, they are asked to sit and pay attention. Children naturally start fidgeting in order to get the movement their body so desperately needs and is not getting enough of to 'turn their brain on.' What happens when the children start fidgeting? We ask them to sit still and pay attention; therefore, their brain goes back to 'sleep.' Therefore, the children are constantly fidgeting and shifting their positions to get comfortable and stabilize themselves.[12]

Clearly, children are not moving nearly enough, and it is resulting in poor core (abdominal) strength and balance. Compared to children from the early 1980s, only 1 out of 12 children has normal strength and balance.[13] More and more children are coming to kindergarten with poor fine motor control. They simply do not have the strength in their hand to utilize the standard tripod grasp of the pencil that allows for efficiency and dexterity when writing. In addition, they may have been given paper-and-pencil activities without sufficient help on proper pencil-holding technique before the appropriate motor areas were ready.[14,15]

Play is important in developing physical strength and motor skills, among other things. But what exactly is play, and how does it make a difference in the way children grow and learn? It turns out that there are different types of play, and research has been done on the benefits they offer. Play is defined as engaging in an activity for enjoyment and recreation rather than a serious or practical purpose.[16] Kids can find enjoyment in many different kinds of recreational activities, including structured, physical activities, like sports, or unstructured activities, like playing ball in the backyard, a board game at the dining room table, or a game of hide and seek. While all of these activities are wonderful experiences for children, they are missing two critical ingredients for the type of play that nurtures a healthy childhood—creativity and imagination. What has been noticeably lacking in the lives of many young children is unstructured, creative, and imaginative play, or free play, as it is sometimes referred to in school settings (although it doesn't happen much anymore). Have you ever observed children engaging in make-believe play? Listen to what they are saying; they engage in what's called private speech. They talk to themselves about what they are going to do and how they are going to do it. It's not just children who use private speech to control themselves. If we look at adults' use of private speech or self-talk, we're often using it to surmount obstacles, to master cognitive and social skills, and to manage our emotions. The more structured the play, the more children's private speech decreases. Creative and imaginative play nurtures brain and body development because:

- It helps to develop the executive control center of the brain, especially self-regulation, focus and attention. Self-regulation is said to be a better predictor of success in life than IQ score. Children who can self-regulate are able to control their attention, impulsivity, and behavior and are better able to control their emotions. The ability to delay gratification in order to achieve long-term goals highly correlates with future success in life.[17]

- It develops gross and fine motor skills and sensory integration.[18]

- It improves social skills because play has a direct impact on "mirror neurons" in the brain, which help us understand intentions and emotions. They help us see the perspectives of others and develop empathy.[19]

- It enhances vocabulary and language skills, which, in turn, will improve reading comprehension and oral and written expression.[20]

- It promotes natural curiosity, creativity, imagination, thinking, and problem solving.

- It improves memory, thinking, decision-making, and speed of mental processing.

- It promotes STEM skills (science, technology, engineering, and math).[21]

- It helps children feel in control of their own lives, which reduces anxiety and depression.[22]

- It increases perseverance, resilience, and coping skills.

- It safely allows children to take risks, learn from mistakes, and strengthen negotiation and leadership skills.

- It allows for practice of real-life situations and prepares children for adulthood.

While anywhere children play is wonderful, playing outside is ideal. Outdoor play provides a natural way to induce chemistry that promotes feelings of euphoria and insulates against depression, anxiety, and stress. It can relieve fatigue and increase creativity.[23] In fact, just a short period of time in the sunlight can raise levels of vitamin D, which helps protect children from future bone problems, heart disease, diabetes, and other health issues.[24]

New research is also showing us that being in natural light or sunlight can have a significant impact on healthy eye development. Over recent decades there has been a significant increase around the globe in short-sightedness, or myopia as it is officially known. It has even reached epidemic levels in East Asia, Singapore, Taiwan, and South Korea, where 90 percent of 18-year-olds are now short-sighted. In Western Europe, about 40 percent to 50 percent of young adults in their mid-20s are short-sighted. In urban China, 10 percent of children in each class per year are becoming short-sighted from about the age of 6. Compare this to research done in Sydney, Australia, that showed only 3 percent of Chinese-heritage children living in Sydney, who spent two hours a day outdoors, were short-sighted by the age of 6, compared to nearly 30 percent of 6-year-olds in Singapore.

Experts have concluded that two hours a day spent in nature seems to be an optimal amount of time to nurture healthy eye development. However, in this day and age, that is difficult to accomplish, especially during the school year.[25] If we, as parents and educators, can make a concerted effort to just increase outdoor time a bit, shouldn't we do that? Perhaps a few more minutes at the bus stop, a walk to school, longer recess, or an outdoor activity (academic, social, or just a "brain break") would allow more time in natural light and a chance for some much needed movement. What about a short playtime or walk outside before tackling homework? Of course, the weekends and summertime provide more opportunities for outdoor play, but given the research and alarming statistics, it would seem that increasing time spent enjoying Mother Nature would be a good idea.

In short, play and playing in nature can affect us in so many positive ways. The importance of free play is well documented, and it plays a significant role in brain development in young children and the improvement of sensory development and to physical and mental health in all individuals.[26]

Fortunately, there are schools in the United States and abroad that understand that play-based learning is the most beneficial way to nurture healthy brain and body development and will yield the most positive outcomes for success in the future. For example, schools in Finland have always believed in the benefits and "power of play," and a typical school day for 6-year-olds starts with an hour of unstructured, outdoor play.[27]

A school in Auckland, New Zealand, has tried a nonconventional, yet successful, approach to recess. Principal Bruce McLachlan changed recess in order to get children grounded, inspired, and ready to learn.[28] By having two 40-minute recesses a day, children are able to have more opportunities to move, explore, and use their imaginations. At recess, children are allowed to climb trees and enjoy bikes, scooters, and loose materials like wooden planks, hoses, and tires—materials that foster imaginative play. Adult supervisors are encouraged to stand back and act as observers rather than facilitators as much as possible, as their philosophy is that children should be encouraged to think creatively and practice independent problem solving.

In the United States, four Texas elementary schools have recently adopted a Finnish model of play and movement-based learning that is structured around four, short recess periods each day. After studying Finland's education system, which consistently scores near the top in international school rankings, Debbie Rhea, associate dean of research and health sciences at Texas Christian University, created the college's Let's Inspire Innovation 'N Kids (LiiNK) program in 2013. In 2015–2016, she began a three-year pilot in two districts in the Fort Worth area. Eagle Mountain Elementary School of the Eagle Mountain-Saginaw ISD in Fort Worth launched LiiNK in fall 2015 for kindergarten and first-grade students and plans to add a grade each upcoming year. Eagle Mountain principal Bryan McLain says, "Kids are not hardwired to sit all day long. This helps give kids back their childhood." Teachers, who were nervous at first, are reporting positive behavioral changes in students and are seeing students who are paying more attention in class, following directions better, attempting to learn more independently, and solving problems on their own.[29]

Several years ago in a local elementary school, the staff started a before school Running Club for third, fourth, and fifth graders. Believe it or not, 58 percent of the students voluntarily come to school two days a week, 40 minutes before school starts, just to be outside. One teacher who sponsors the activity told me, "We get the runners, the joggers, the walkers, and the strollers. They race each other, talk with their friends, explore plant and insect life, sit at the picnic tables, and play on the wooden train. They just enjoy the outdoors for 40 uninterrupted, unmanaged (though lightly supervised) minutes. Younger students often show up with their parents and just enjoy

being on the nature trail that adjoins the playground."
While there has been no formal data to track the behavior
and academic performance of the "running-club kids"
and the "non-running-club kids," some of the teachers feel
that the club has had a positive effect on the participants.

—Perk

Recess used to be and should still be a time to relax and play. It should be a time to be in nature, interact with the environment, and perhaps even dig in the dirt under the shade of a tree. It's a time to talk with friends, develop gross and fine motor skills, nurture one's creativity and imagination, and be rejuvenated to go back into the classroom and engage in other academic pursuits. Recess shouldn't be such a challenge for children that school counselors have to design "alternate recesses" with structured games and activities for children who have difficulty navigating the social world of the playground. It shouldn't require school districts to hire companies that specialize in facilitating recess activities and teaching social skills.[30, 31] However, this is the reality in many school settings that don't embrace a play-based approach to education. Despite the rigors of challenging curriculums and state testing, many dedicated and caring teachers who value and understand the importance of play and hands-on learning activities have found their own creative ways to incorporate old-fashioned play and skill building, and developmentally appropriate activities into the school day.

In the summer of 2007, a group of my colleagues and
I gathered for our annual trip to the shore. As we sat
around lamenting the loss of play and the increase in
behavior problems in the classroom, the idea of an ICE
room was born. Imaginative, Creative, Exploration—a
room where kids could be kids and still learn at the
same time. The room was designed with the help of our
instructional support team members and occupational

therapists. Our very supportive principal and wonderful Parent Teacher Organization donated funds. Every week the kindergarteners, pre-firsters, and first graders are able to go to the ICE room and engage in all those activities that they don't get to do anymore. In addition, many of the center activities are designed to strengthen fine motor skills and nurture a proper pencil grip. Because of the amount of work it takes to plan and organize the materials and activities and the limited time in the room, the children are told that there is "zero tolerance" of inappropriate or disruptive behavior. There are no warnings. Any children who cannot follow the ICE room rules will be "uninvited" and asked to leave the room. I think in the 10 years that the room has been in existence, only one or two children have been excused, and they were only excused once. They learned their lesson and were on their best behavior from then on. Year after year the ICE room continues to be a favorite place for students and teachers.

—Perk

Although there are many activities that are rotated through the ICE room month after month, by far the most favorite—every year—is the vet center. Children pretend to be veterinarians and pet owners as they play with a variety of stuffed animals and real supplies like stethoscopes, dog crates, leashes, bandages, file folders, and calendars, etc. Once this center is introduced, the children never want it taken away! The other all-time favorites are what I consider "old fashioned" toys: playdough, wooden building blocks, toy cars on a floor road mat, and games such as Operation, Topple, Perfection, and Light Bright. We actually choose games that enhance fine motor strength but are fun to play. These games are a novelty to the children who have been entertained and raised with electronic games. They love going to the ICE room.

—Kathy Newell, first-grade teacher

Due to a lack of creative, imaginative, and unstructured play, the mental and physical health of several generations of children has been impacted. It has taken many years for parents, educators, and researchers to become aware of these negative consequences and to voice their concerns. Children can't always advocate for themselves, so we, as parents and educators, must create change and speak for them. We are hopeful that the pendulum is swinging back as more voices cry out for a return to a world where children can unleash their creativity and imagination and just play. In chapter 9, we offer many ideas and strategies to foster active and creative play!

Tips for Bringing Back Play

Tip 1. Playing with your children can help them learn how to play. Building with blocks, engaging in imaginative role-playing, or building castles in the sand is all that it will take to help nurture their creativity.

Tip 2. Invite family and neighbors over for a get together and encourage the kids to just play—in a sandbox, on the swing set, in a tent (or a big box or table with a blanket over it), or gather together random materials for building and see what happens.

Tip 3. When possible, seek out preschools and daycares that are play-based and allow for time spent in creative, imaginative play—inside and outside.

In chapter 9, we offer additional ideas and strategies to help families engage in more play opportunities.

Chapter six

The Hidden Dangers of Screen Time

"Technology should improve your life . . . Not become your life."

—Billy Cox

Technology has taken our world by storm. If you buy a device one day, it's almost outdated the next. Television has allowed us to watch man walk on the moon, presidents be sworn into office, weddings of royalty, funerals of dignitaries, breaking news, and provided entertainment in the comfort of our own homes. Computers and other technologies allow us to easily stay in touch with family and friends and access information about any given topic, and assistive technology is a godsend for those with disabilities. Businesses, educational institutions, and the medical world rely on technology to improve efficiency, communication, services, instruction, and health. It has simplified our lives, and it has complicated our lives at the same time—it can be a blessing and a curse. Like anything, moderation and balance are key. Let's take a look at what happens when the world of technology becomes unbalanced.

"I think he should pick Becca. She's pretty." "No, I think he should pick Whitney. She's a nurse. I want to be a nurse." Suddenly I realized what I was hearing. This was a conversation between two first-grade girls the morning after an episode of The Bachelor (yes, I was watching it, too, but I am a grown-up). They went on to give all their reasons for why he should "dump" one woman and give a rose to the other. On another occasion, a kindergartener accompanied her parent to an R-rated movie and came to school the next day sharing the language and mature scenes with her classmates. Too young to know better, she spared no detail and spoke about scenes that were sexual and violent in nature as if they were commonplace. As educators, we've noticed that more and more young children are staying up too late and watching shows and movies that are not meant for them. For these students and others, the exposure to entertainment meant for adults has no boundaries and normalizes any behaviors they witness.

Another example of screen time gone awry concerns an adorable first grader named Nathan. I gave him a note for his mom, and he said, "She won't read it." When I asked him why, he told me, "She is always on her phone." Before I knew it, I was brainstorming with a 6-year-old about where he could leave the note so that Mommy would be sure to see and read it. I mentioned her place at the kitchen table. "No, that won't work. We don't eat at the table." Later, when I shared this story with Mom, she admitted that she is always on the phone. And yes, I witnessed it for several years to come. Even at holiday concerts and other family events at school, her children and many others were competing with their parents' cell phones. Whether it is business-imposed or self-imposed accountability, it's not easy for adults to put down their phones, disconnect, and relax. Given that 1 in 10 people is genetically predisposed toward addictive tendencies, it's easy to see how individuals can become "hooked," if not addicted, to screen time.[1] In the absence of connections with parents or other family members, disconnected children can easily attach to devices instead.

—*Perk*

An anecdote from the article "*It's 'Digital Heroin': How Screens Turn Kids into Psychotic Junkies*" by Dr. Nicholas Kardaras highlights the type of behavior that can result when children have too much screen time: John was a 6-year-old boy whose mother, Susan, bought him an iPad. Susan began letting John play educational games, and one day he discovered Minecraft. Susan began to see changes in her son that were alarming. He became more engrossed in the game and lost interest in other activities that he used to enjoy. He refused to do his chores and reported seeing game images in his dreams. As his behavior began to deteriorate, she tried to take the game away, but John demonstrated severe behavior outbursts. They were so severe, his mother just gave in and allowed him to play more Minecraft. Then one night, she knew John had a serious problem. He was sitting up in his bed staring wide-eyed as if in a trance as his glowing iPad lay next to him on the bed. She had to shake him repeatedly to snap him out of a catatonic stupor.[2]

Or consider the quote from another child, Athena: "I would rather be on my phone in my room watching Netflix than spending time with my family . . . I think we like our phones more than we like actual people."[3]

Let's be real. Technology is here to stay, and we all use some type of screen every day. However, the research, data, and personal observations tell us that too much screen time can negatively affect many aspects of our physical and mental health, and it's so loud and clear that we cannot ignore it.[4, 5] The following sections highlight areas of our life that are impacted by screen time.

Impact on Brain Development

- Screen time can cause a release of dopamine, the "feel good" chemical or neurotransmitter. Remember that these neurotransmitters exist in a careful balance that allows us to carry out cognitive and learning-oriented tasks. If the careful balance is disturbed by the overuse of technology, as studies are beginning to show, one might expect to see problems that impact mood, behavior, attention, and learning.[6]

- It can cause one's brain to shrink, as volume is lost in the area that controls impulses (striatum). It can also cause changes in the regions of the brain that are involved in emotional processing, decision-making, and thought control.

- It can damage the brain's insular cortex, the region where compassion, social cues, and emotions are developed.[7]

- It can cause a lack of development in the frontal lobe where the "executive function" systems are located (prioritizing, planning, focusing, inhibiting impulsivity, self-regulation, delaying gratification, and empathy).[8]

- It can cause damage to the brain's white matter, leading to a breakdown between thinking and surviving.[9] (Recall the upstairs and downstairs brain example in chapter 2.)

Impact on Attention and Behavior

- Too much screen time can reduce "stick-to-it-ness."

- It can cause fragmented attention. Children frequently look away from TV for "reduction of stimulation."[10] They are usually drawn back by special effects, which then encourages the future need for the equivalent of "special effects" in the classroom in order to maintain attention.

- It can create a passive withdrawal or "zombie effect," with much less active brain wave activity than when reading a book.

When it comes to engaging in screen time in the car, authors of the article, "Smartphones Are Killing Americans—But Nobody Is Counting," say that "the problem of 'death by distraction' has gotten much worse." After decades of declining deaths on the road, U.S. traffic fatalities surged by 14.4 percent between 2014 and 2016. The increase doesn't seem to be explained away by an increase in speeding, drinking, or more driving. More alarming is that this increase in deaths includes more pedestrian, bicyclist, and motorcycle fatalities. What does coincide with the surge of vehicular deaths is the substantial increase in smartphone use by U.S. drivers as they drive. From 2014 to 2016, the share of Americans who owned a mobile phone increased from 75 percent to 81 percent, with motorists speaking on the phone more while driving instead of watching the road.[11]

When attention suffers, so does the ability to process one's internal and external worlds, which can wreak havoc on healthy development.[12]

Impact on the Body

- Too much screen time can reduce fine and gross motor development and can increase obesity due to the sedentary nature of viewing.[13]

- It results in overstimulation to the sympathetic nervous system, causing hyperarousal, elevated adrenalin, and an eventual rise in cortisol, significantly increasing risk for heart attacks and strokes.[14] In addition, when children are in a constant state of high arousal, they may seem "wired and tired." These chronic states of high arousal negatively affect mood, memory, and the ability to relate to others. These children may exhibit behaviors that resemble and actually result in a mental health diagnosis that may, in fact, not be warranted. The good news is that time spent in nature can restore focus, lower stress, and reduce aggression.[15]

- Sending multiple texts a day can cause inflammation in your fingers, leading to tendinitis, arthritis, or "trigger finger," a condition that causes fingers to get stuck in a bent position.[16] Surgery can be required to fix this condition.

- 90 percent of us text with our necks bent, which strains muscles, tendons, and ligaments. Flexing the neck forward at a 60-degree angle puts 60 pounds of weight on the spine, leading to degeneration and arthritis.[17] Many chiropractors are now seeing patients of all ages with "text neck."

- 65 percent of Americans suffer from digital eye strain, a condition characterized by dry, itchy eyes and blurred vision. Narrowed blood vessels in eyes have been noted as a result of too much screen time with unknown long-term effects. The blue light emitted by most smartphones may damage the retina, leading to macular degeneration.[18]

- Increased hours in front of screens may account for the rise in the number of children who are near-sighted and/or have reading difficulties that have a visual component.[19]

- Too much screen time can negatively impact sleep.[20]

The Kaiser Foundation reports that 75 percent of children aged 9 and 10 are sleep deprived.[21] In addition to watching TV or using a computer or smart device, nighttime light exposure from the high-intensity light on the screens of these devices scrambles and disrupts the body's circadian rhythms, which evolved to follow the cycles of natural daylight and affect sleep cycles by influencing the body's production of melatonin. Over time, chronic fatigue sets in, causing a myriad of physical and mental health issues. Some research has shown that a lack of sleep "may" contribute to cancer, diabetes, heart disease, and obesity. It is critical for the body to get to a REM sleep cycle, because it is during REM sleep that the brain consolidates memories and the day's learning.[22]

According to one theory, sleep is the brain's overnight rinse cycle, a time for flushing the cellular debris generated by metabolic activity. Charles Czeisler, chief of the Division of Sleep and Circadian Disorders at Brigham and Women's Hospital in Boston, states, "The brain has to go offline during that process. That's what we call sleep."[23] In addition, when children go to sleep while viewing a movie or TV show, the content may be disturbing and cause nightmares, which can also disrupt REM sleep. Suffice it to say, a plethora of negative effects can result from not running your "neurochemical dishwasher." One bad night can translate into a day of diminished executive function, foggy memory, and sludgy mental acuity. In older adults, it can also speed the development of cognitive impairment. For students, the next school day may be challenging and not very productive.[24]

Another side effect of too much screen time is increased exposure to radiation. Exposure to radiation can cause debilitating and severe physical and mental health issues. We would be remiss if we didn't offer a particular word of caution for negative health outcomes when using cell phones and other wireless devices. In May of 2011, the World Health Organization classified cell phones and other wireless devices as a category 2B risk (possible carcinogen) due to radiation emission. James McNamee with Health Canada in October of 2011 issued a cautionary warning stating, "Children are more sensitive to a variety of agents than adults as their brains and immune systems are still developing, so you can't say the risk would be equal for a small adult as for a child." In December 2013, Dr. Anthony Miller from the University of Toronto's School of Public Health recommended that based on new research, radio-frequency exposure should be reclassified as a 2A (probable carcinogen), not a 2B (possible carcinogen).[25] The American Academy of Pediatrics (AAP) has requested a review of EMF radiation emissions from technology devices. As radiation standards are reassessed, the AAP has urged the FCC to adopt radiation standards that protect children's health and well-being, reflect current use patterns, and provide meaningful consumer disclosure.[26]

If we were asked you how much more radiation penetrates your body today versus 10 years ago, what would you say? According to Olle Johansson, a professor of neuroscience in Sweden, it is a quintillion times more—that is a one with 18 zeros! Because of the overwhelming concern about the effects of this radiation, especially on young children, France has done away with wireless Internet in elementary schools because wired computers do not expose the children to radio-frequency radiation. What are some sources of this radiation? Microwaves, cell phones and other devices (especially when placed directly on your body), wireless Internet networks, and smart boxes, which are digital meters that are being installed by utility companies nationwide to measure energy usage are just a few examples.[27] Smart meters can overexpose the general population to high frequencies, which can be potentially dangerous for everyone, especially with long-term usage. However, for a small percentage of the population, about 3 percent to 15 percent, it can be debilitating and cause severe physical and mental health issues immediately. This group suffers from radio-frequency sickness, sometimes called electromagnetic hypersensitivity (EHS). Some experts estimate that continued long-term exposure could increase that percentage to 50 percent in five years. The good news is that "radio frequency sickness is not a disease. It is an environmental induced functional impairment." Eliminate the source and hopefully, the symptoms will go with it![28]

Impact on Social and Emotional Development

- Too much screen time can inhibit emotional development in young children and can impact adults, too.[29]

- It can normalize violence and can increase aggression.

- It can encourage provocative and/or premature sexual behavior.

- It encourages the brain to seek the unique and different, that is, novelty. There can be a dark side to this increased novelty-seeking behavior, especially in the teenage years.

- Teens who spend more time on social media are less likely to be involved in or value community and are less interested in news and current events.[30]

- It encourages social anonymity, disconnectedness, and feelings of sadness and hopelessness.

- It can discourage the natural development of social skills.

- It can discourage the natural development of empathy.

As recently as the year 2000, every G-rated movie contained violence, as did 60 percent of prime time television shows. In 1998, it was estimated that the typical child would have seen 8,000 murders and 100,000 other acts of violence, including rape and assault, before middle school. These figures are limited to television. Today's children experience screen violence on many different devices. Therefore, media researchers and pediatricians refer to children's "media diets" as a way of communicating the amount and type of viewing that is consumed. Like food diets, media diets can be healthy or unhealthy, balanced or unbalanced, with moderation of consumption being key.[31]

Suicide rates have increased in recent years. After declining over a 20-year period, an increase in suicide rates among U.S. teens occurred from 2009 to 2015—this was the same time that social media usage surged. A recent study has suggested that there may be a link. Teens' use of electronic devices, including smartphones, for at least five hours daily more than doubled, from 8 percent in 2009 to 19 percent in 2015. These teens were 70 percent more likely to have suicidal thoughts or actions than those who reported one hour of daily use.[32] In two national surveys of U.S. adolescents in grades 8–12, adolescents who spent more time on nonscreen activities (i.e., face-to-face interactions, sports, exercise, print media, and attendance at religious services) were less likely to have mental health issues.[33]

Today's teens (coined the iGeneration by author Jean Twenge) tend to stay at home and connect with friends on social media.

They actually see their friends an hour less a day than their generation predecessors (Gen Xers and early Millennials), which is an hour less a day of building communication and social skills and negotiating relationships.[34]

When people hide behind a screen, as they can when using social media, they cannot see the reactions from others when they say something unkind, which is so important for developing empathy. Recent teen suicides have been blamed on cyberbullying and social media comparisons made between oneself and others' posts depicting the "perfect" life and friends. Dr. Victor Strasburger, a teen medicine specialist at the University of New Mexico, states, "With its immediacy, anonymity, and potential for bullying, social media has a unique potential for causing real harm."[35]

Anna Dewdney, author of many children's books, wrote a 2013 opinion piece for the *Wall Street Journal*, emphasizing that when it comes to educating children "empathy is as important as literacy." She wrote:

> When we open a book and share our voice and imagination with a child, that child learns to see the world through someone else's eyes. We are doing something that I believe is just as powerful, and it is something that we are losing as a culture: by reading with a child, we are teaching that child to be human.[36]

Impact on Language Development

Too much screen time can affect language development, both in verbal and written expression. According to Jane Healy, author of *Endangered Minds: Why Children Can't Think—and What We Can Do About It*, children are developing a "McLanguage" of sorts. Children come to school with a deficient base for higher-order language and reasoning skills. They are not speaking properly because they don't hear the words pronounced slowly. Spelling is declining because they don't hear the sounds. Grammar skills and basic concepts are weak. Vocabulary is weak, but understanding of more mature, and at times, inappropriate vocabulary may be present. Many learning disabilities are rooted in language delays, and yet children are permitted to be "linguistically malnourished."[37] Increasing the number of vocabulary words that children hear and know and improving their ability to visualize concepts and symbols are critical skills to future reading success.[38] In fact, learning to speak more than one language can be beneficial in many ways, including improved communication skills, better memory, stronger executive functioning skills, a heightened awareness for other cultures, and increased empathy.[39] Too much screen time can also negatively impact listening and communication skills, which has a trickle-down effect on phonological awareness and reading and spelling skill development overall.

Impact on Spelling and Reading

With more children growing up texting, the use of abbreviations and unconventional spelling increases, and for some it's hard to differentiate when it's okay to communicate informally versus formally (i.e., correct/full spelling of words and proper grammar). Spending more time in front a screen has also led to less joyful and less proficient readers. Evidence suggests that children who read exclusively on-screen are three times less likely to say they enjoy reading, a third less likely to have a favorite book, and far less likely to be strong readers.[40] Furthermore, having too much screen time can cause trouble with comprehension or more difficult reading material with longer sentences, embedded clauses, and more advanced grammatical structures. Dr. John S. Hutton, a clinical research fellow at Cincinnati Children's Hospital Medical Center, reported that when older children read to themselves, there is a significantly greater activation of the brain's left hemisphere, which if you recall from chapter 2, is where the brain works with words. What we also know is that this part of the brain lights up when younger children are hearing stories. The children can imagine in their mind's eye and visualize what the characters look like and what they are doing. We tell the children that it is like "making a movie in your mind." A memory that you can "see" is a memory that you can find when trying to remember details about a story or answer comprehension questions.[41]

In her book *UnSelfie: Why Empathetic Kids Succeed in Our All About Me World*, author Michele Borba addresses the issue about reading and screen time and shares the following alarming statistics:[42]

- 45 percent of 17-year-olds admit they read by choice only once or twice a year.

- Parents are reading to their children less and less, and yet we know that it is important that young children hear language, and that they need to hear it from people, not from screens. In 1999, children aged 2 to 7 years were read to for an average of 45 minutes a day. In 2013, that number dropped to just over 30 minutes a day.

- Only 64 percent of parents say they read bedtime stories to their children, although 90 percent said they did when their children were young.

- More than half of kids said they preferred watching television to reading. As digital entertainment choices rise, Borba predicts that our kids' reading habits will continue to decline.

Reading on a screen is different than reading a handheld book. Technology writer Nicholas Carr explains that reading a book is like scuba diving in which the diver is submerged in a quiet, slow-paced setting without distractions. This allows the diver or reader to focus and think deeply about the information in the book. Compare this to using the Internet, which he compares to jet skiing. The jet skier (i.e., the reader) is skimming along the surface at a high speed and frequently hops over the surface. There are many distractions, which results in limited focus on any one thing. Finally, reading develops critical-thinking ability, problem-solving skills, and vocabulary better than visual media.

In a 2003 study, nearly 80 percent of 687 surveyed students preferred to read text on paper as opposed to on a screen in order to "understand it with clarity." For young children, interactive books, or "e-books," have been linked to lower levels of story understanding and may hinder aspects of emergent literacy.[43]

Think about what a screen looks like when the news is on. On what do you focus? The trailer at the bottom of the TV screen? What the anchorman is saying? The graphics being projected on the screen? This is a perfect example of fragmented attention and only comprehending bits and pieces of several topics. On the computer or other device, the news comes across in headlines, small snippets, and hyperlinks. Many people read just that part and not the entire article, again affecting their comprehension of the "big picture." As they get older, students need to learn to extend their ability to focus and read more deeply on a given topic. It's not impossible to do that on a screen, but it is more physically and mentally taxing than reading on paper.

Impact on Writing Ability

Spending an excess of time on front of a screen can reduce understanding and memory for new material. Despite living in the world of technology, teaching students an efficient means of writing still has merit. Remember from chapter 2, there is an important region of our brain called the occipitotemporal cortex where visual stimuli actually become letters and written words. You have to be able to visualize the letters in order to remember how to write them on paper. Brain imaging shows that the activation of this region is different in children who are having trouble with handwriting. Children who have trouble with handwriting may also have trouble becoming efficient and successful readers.[44] In addition, printing and cursive writing stimulate the brain in areas such as eye-hand coordination, attention to detail, thinking, language, and working memory skills. When students take notes by hand, their understanding of and memory for the material are greatly improved compared to using a laptop computer for note taking. One brave college professor at South Texas College of Law advocated for banning laptops in the classroom. He presented much evidence supporting his ban, and in the end nearly 90 percent of his students reported feeling positive or neutral about the keyboard ban. The professor noted more interaction and participation from his students and higher exams scores, too.[45]

With the increased presence of technology in schools, there is a lack of focus on mastering an efficient system of writing, be it manuscript or cursive. Some parents and educators believe that kids should just be taught keyboarding skills and not worry about writing by hand. After all, they can always type on a keyboard. Educators who have been in the trenches for many years would tell you this is not a wise move. Consider the following:

> *The reality is that for decades, students in most elementary schools were taught to print during kindergarten, first grade, and second grade. Much to the delight of most students, cursive was (and in some schools still is) introduced in the second grade. It continued to be taught, reinforced, and required through fifth grade. By the time students went on to sixth or seventh grade, they were fluent and efficient writers and note takers. Now they could focus on the content and mechanics of their writing. For the last 10 years or so, this is not the case. Handwriting instruction is "hit or miss" depending on the district's curriculum and the teachers' philosophy of its importance. For the most part, the art of handwriting, manuscript or cursive, is a dying art. This presents a problem because now many students have not mastered one efficient*

system of writing. Their printing is haphazard with many of the letters or numerals being formed incorrectly and inefficiently, and in some cases the writing is illegible. They typically try to write the bare minimum because it's tiresome and laborious. When kids start using any electronic device's keyboard at an early age, they may not have the fine motor skills to master efficient keyboarding skills and tend to use the "hunt and peck" method or just use one finger on each hand. Again, this is not an efficient or fast method for note taking or communication.

You might want to try this experiment with your child or maybe even do it yourself. Fold a paper into thirds. Rather than timing each of the following three activities for 1 minute, do 30 seconds, and then you can multiply your results by two to save time. In the first box, have your child make vertical strokes from the bottom up for 30 seconds. Repeat in the second box for 30 seconds but this time alternate strokes from the bottom up and then top down. In the third box for 30 seconds make vertical marks from the top down. Count the number of strokes in each and multiply by two. That is the number of strokes per minute. See which sample—1, 2, or 3—has more strokes and the neatest, most consistent strokes. It's usually the third box because this is the correct way to form manuscript letters—from the top down. Today, most kids draw their letters or start at the bottom, which discourages neatness and reduces efficiency.

In the last 10 to 15 years, I get many more referrals that center around writing. Sometimes the concern is due to difficulties expressing and organizing one's thoughts. Sometimes it's due to not having a "formula" for constructing sentences. Those weaknesses can be remediated with direct, systematic instruction. However, almost always, there is also a fine motor or handwriting component. It could be an inefficient pencil grip, a lack

*of correct letter or numeral formation, difficulties utiliz-
ing lines and spaces, or all of the above. Of course, the
earlier the intervention, the easier it is to undo the bad
habits. However, after a few years of an awkward pencil
grip and incorrect formations, it is almost impossible for
the student to want to make a change or even be able to
do so. In that case, teaching a new system that hasn't
been used is an option, because no bad habits have been
developed. Accuracy, fluency, efficiency, and legibility can
be greatly improved, thus allowing more focus on the
content and mechanics of writing. However, learning any
new task requires daily practice and dedication, and for
handwriting this is hard to achieve in a weekly tutoring
session outside of the school day.*

—Perk

Virginia Berninger, a professor of educational psychology
at the University of Washington, said the research suggests that
children need introductory training in printing, then two years of
learning and practicing cursive, starting in grade three, and then
some systematic attention to touch-typing. "What we're advocat-
ing is teaching children to be hybrid writers," said Dr. Berninger,
"manuscript first for reading—it transfers to better word recognition—then cursive for spelling and for composing. Then, starting in
late elementary school, touch-typing."[46] Interestingly, this is exactly
what was done so successfully for many years.

Impact on Learning

If the declining rates of reading books/printed material still allowed
teens to keep up with their academic skills, there might not be
cause for concern. However, SAT scores have declined since the
mid-2000s, especially in writing, where there has been a 13-point

decline since 2006. In critical reading, there has been a 13-point decline since 2005. Math scores have also declined, but still remain higher than reading and writing scores. As stated earlier, reading comprehension and academic writing skills are declining, which may be due to short attention spans that the new media encourages. One study revealed that students working on their computers switched between tasks every 19 seconds on average. More than 75 percent of students' computer windows were open less than one minute. This is very different than sitting and reading a book for hours and has posed a challenge for educators, especially at the high school and college levels, because they're unsure how students are going to digest the typical multipage textbook or required reading. Many students simply don't read the material, which has caused publishers to move toward more interactive e-books to try and keep their students engaged, shorter books that are more conversational in writing style, and video sharing.[47]

We believe that parents and educators have always known that reading, spelling, and writing are important factors for academic success. Any educator of young children will tell you that it is absolutely critical that students be fluent and successful readers by fourth grade. After that, it becomes more difficult to remediate reading, spelling, and writing skills to grade-level benchmarks. As their education continues, students will be reading to learn, not learning to read. Reading and writing requirements will increase and without fluent skills, schoolwork and homework will become laborious and frustrating, and long-term success in academics and eventually career may be affected.

The Technology Dilemma

More and more adults are using computers and iPads with children from a very early age in an attempt to assist with learning. However, no credible evidence exists that any type of screen time is beneficial to babies and toddlers and, in fact, there is some evidence that it may be harmful.[48] Many times, as students enter school, technology has its place. It can be a godsend for some students, and for others it is the "hook" that is needed to get them invested in their schoolwork. Technology can also be used to help with implementation of accommodations and interventions for students with special needs and simplify communication and tracking of behavior.

What seems to be happening in the United States is that companies have effectively convinced school districts into believing that electronic devices in daycares, preschools, and elementary schools are somehow critical and educational.[49] School districts nationwide have loaded up students with tablets, iPods, laptops, and more so that they are prepared to compete with students around the globe. Some teachers expect all work from students to be submitted via technology (Chromebooks, computers, etc.), and school administrators expect teachers to use the electronic components of the adopted curriculum. Suffice it to say, in some cases this means a great deal of instruction and school work are carried out via a smartboard or other electronic device beginning in kindergarten.

In other countries, technology is used, but at much lower usage rates than the United States. Other countries prefer instead to provide young learners with what their young brains need to develop. In Finland, students and teachers don't need laptops and iPads to get to the top of international education rankings. Officials say they aren't interested in using them to stay there. The Nordic country uses innovative teaching strategies in the classroom, generally without incorporating technology, and still Finnish students have repeatedly outperformed American students on international tests.[50]

Perhaps one might think that there is a bigger focus on technology in education in China. Formal technology education begins in third grade, but the use of technology in school is minimal, and students rarely use a computer to type reports or for writing assignments. In addition, computer addiction is a major worry for parents and teachers in China. China's Ministry of Health is conducting research on Internet addiction, which is termed "pathological internet use." Guo Dazhong, assistant director of computer education in the state-run Jingan District Youth Center in Shanghai, states, "How to solve the addiction to online games is a big challenge." Guo goes on to say, "Kids are naturally drawn to computers. Other countries also face similar issues."[51]

Even famous tech designers, engineers, and social media executives like Steve Jobs and Tim Cook (Apple), Bill Gates (Microsoft), Mark Zuckerberg and Sean Parker (Facebook), and Jack Dorsey and Ned Segal (Twitter) have openly shared they are tech-cautious parents. These social media executives are simply following the rule of drug pushers and dealers everywhere, "Never get high on your own supply."[52,53] This is probably why many employees of eBay, Apple, Yahoo!, and Hewlett-Packard opt to send their children to a Waldorf School, which believes in a more simplistic and retro approach to education and no technology until about eighth grade. Classrooms are equipped with blackboards, colored chalk, real books (including encyclopedias), desks, and #2 pencils. The feeling is that these students will have no trouble catching up to the world of technology. One parent, who holds a computer science degree from Dartmouth and works at Google, states, "At Google and all these places, we make technology as brain-dead easy to use as possible. There's no reason why kids can't figure it out when they get older." As Bill Gates says, "Technology is just a tool. In terms of getting the kids working together and motivating them, the teacher is the most important." Even shareholders of Apple, Inc. are concerned about addictive qualities and harmful effects of the iPhone that could hurt children and want the company to study the effects of heavy usage on mental health.[54]

Screen Addiction

Watching television shows and movies on screens is not new. Some of you might be thinking, "We watched a lot of TV when we were kids, and we're OK. So what's the big deal about screen time now?" The problem is television is qualitatively different than the new generation of technology. Television is passive stimulation. In the past, prior to DVR and "on demand" features, when a show was over, so was the screen time. Families typically had one TV, and there was usually an adult nearby to monitor the content and amount of viewing time.

That is not the case in homes today where there may be televisions and other screens in many rooms of the home, including children's bedrooms and even in the family car. Today's televisions are very different and have many bells and whistles, including split screens for viewing multiple shows or sporting events. Over the years, programming has dramatically changed to include darker themes and no limit to sex, violence, and bad language. Storylines have changed from a one-line plot with a beginning, middle, and an end to shows with multiple storylines. Consider the popularity of shows like *24* and *Game of Thrones*, which masterfully keep the viewer thinking about many things at once. Why have the shows' writers taken this approach? Perhaps, it's because attention spans became shorter, and viewers needed the variety and stimulation of multiple plots and storylines to stay engaged.

Whether viewing something on TV or another electronic device, it's very easy to get "lost" in an interesting show or movie to the point that you don't even hear your name being called. However, a TV show or movie has a time limit and then it's over. It's easier to get lost in screen time activities on the computer, smartphone, or tablet because there is no limit to the amount of time you can be on the device. Have you ever been online reading or researching articles or communicating with friends on social media and realized that hours had passed by? Ned Hallowell, author and renowned psychiatrist, refers to this as "screen sucking."[55] One link leads you to an article with an embedded link that leads you elsewhere, and before you know it you are knee deep in a website and have no idea how you got there. Researchers at the University College London have found that the brain's senses of vision and hearing share a limited processing capacity, so the brain is often forced to choose between them. They literally may not hear you calling. Rather than demonstrating "selective hearing," the person you are trying to speak to may be suffering from "inattentional deafness."[56] Modern interactive tablets, game boxes, and handheld devices are much more immersive and interactive than the passive stimulation of television. The radiant screen itself has a very hypnotic effect on children, making it much like a digital drug, therefore making it much easier to get lost in and even addicted to screens.[57]

Video games and online gaming are other sources that can suck you in. On a positive note, many games are creative, educational, and promote problem-solving and analytical thinking. They might even challenge you to wrestle with ethical or moral dilemmas and provide intellectual stimulation. One 2008 study found that video game playing was linked to increased visual memory, while another paper that same year reported that gamers scored higher than the general population on vision, hearing, and spatial ability tests.[58] In the town of Celebration, Florida, surgeons prepare for surgery by playing a few minutes of a video game that is conveniently available in the surgical lounge. "Minimally invasive surgery is ultimately the most important video game in the world," said Dr. Jay Redan, general surgeon at Florida Hospital Celebration Health. "We do all of our work looking at a television screen. Warm-up and practice before operating on someone should be considered as an addition to a surgeon's pre-op preparation routine."[59] Suffice it to say, that certain video games, when played in moderation, have provided a positive contribution to society.

However, educationally oriented games are receiving competition from games that allow the player to become immersed in another world that can provide an alternate reality. Video gaming is a lucrative field that can be exploited for monetary gains. Consequently, those kinds of games are attracting game designers who are driven by the almighty dollar. Video designers want players to keep playing, and they make their games just difficult enough to be challenging, while allowing the player small rewards to keep them engaged, not all that different a concept from gambling casinos that allow players to have small rewards to keep them playing.[60,61] Eventually, some individuals, including children, cannot pull away and are not able to function well in their lives.

In 2008, countries such as China, South Korea, and Japan categorized Internet addiction as a mental illness. Japan is presently reporting a 60 percent technology addiction rate in their youth and has started educating children about technology addictions as early as kindergarten.[62] However, it was not recognized as a problem or disorder in the United States until May 2013 when "Internet Use Disorder" was added to the American Psychiatric Association's *Diagnostic and Statistical Manual of Mental Health Disorders* (DSM-V).[63]

The research is clear that the overuse of screens can negatively and seriously impact brain development and alter physical and mental health. Dr. Nicholas Kardaras, executive director of The Dunes East Hampton, one of the country's top rehabs and author of *Glow Kids: How Screen Addiction Is Hijacking Our Kids—and How to Break the Trance*, states:

> We now know that those iPads, Smartphones and Xboxes are a form of digital drug. Recent brain imaging research is showing that they affect the brain's frontal cortex—which controls executive functioning, including impulse control—in exactly the same way that cocaine does. Technology is so hyper-arousing that it raises dopamine levels—the feel-good neurotransmitter most involved in the addiction dynamic.[64]

This addictive effect is why Dr. Peter Whybrow, director of neuroscience at UCLA, calls screens "electronic cocaine," and Chinese researchers call them "digital heroin." In fact, Dr. Andrew Doan, the head of addiction research for the Pentagon and the U.S. Navy, who has been researching video game addiction, calls video games and screen technologies "digital pharmakeia" (Greek for "drug").[65] Dr. Doan reports that the University of Washington uses video gaming as a tool to numb pain. While playing a virtual game called *Snowworld*, patients release enough endorphins and are visually distracted to a point that nurses can scrub and treat the burns in pediatric and adult patients. When individuals are in front of screens, they can appear numb and oblivious, and it is like "putting them on an IV drip of morphine."[66] Video gaming also relieves the symptoms of psychological pain and can serve as an escape for many children who are experiencing feelings of loneliness, low self-esteem, or stress surrounding school and/or family life.

If you are wondering what ever happened to 6-year-old John (mentioned earlier in the chapter), his mother (a client of Dr. Kardaras) removed John's tablet and accessed professional support from Dr. Kardaras who states that the prescribed amount of time to reset a hyperaroused nervous system is four to six weeks. That's no easy task when screens are everywhere. A person can live without drugs or alcohol; with tech addiction, digital temptations are everywhere. Recovery from any addiction can be an uphill battle with many setbacks along the way. Four years later, after much support, John is doing much better. He is using a desktop computer and has gotten some sense of balance back in his life.[67]

Why is it that so many people can't seem to stay off their phones or other electronic devices? Psychologist Jocelyn Brewer says, "Screen time stimulates happy chemicals like dopamine in the brain." Dopamine is a mood-regulating hormone associated with feelings of pleasure. Brewer says, "It works similarly to other addictions in that there is a reward pathway that dopamine sets up. If you are doing something that feels good, you are going to want to do more of it."[68] What researchers are finding is that external stimulation such as that received by playing video games, can alter the balance of neurotransmitters. This idea is substantiated by a study in 2005 at Hammersmith Hospital in London which found the levels of dopamine in video game players' brains actually doubled while they were playing games.[69] In this case, it is believed that there is actually a physiological brain chemistry change that occurs, causing a possible addiction. A psychological addiction also can occur because video games are designed to be "addictive."

Not only is video gaming addictive, but cell phone and Internet usage has become a serious physical and mental health problem. So how much time do high school seniors spend online, gaming, and texting? A lot, according to Jean Twenge, author of *iGen: Why*

Today's Super-Connected Kids Are Growing Up Less Rebellious, More Tolerant, Less Happy—and Completely Unprepared for Adulthood, who reports the following data (on average):[70]

- Two and a quarter hours a day texting on their cell phones

- Two hours a day on the Internet

- One and a half hours a day on electronic gaming

- Half an hour on video chat

That totals about six hours a day on screens. Eighth graders were not far behind, and there was not much difference in usage based on family background. Subtract that from 24 hours, and you are left with 18 hours. Teens typically spend 17 hours a day in school, sleeping, and on homework and extracurricular activities. That leaves about one hour for some TV viewing, although the data says that teens typically watch two hours a day. Chances are they are probably multitasking and/or sleeping less, which we have pointed out to be concerns for healthy development.

Brain development takes time, and most brains are not fully developed until the age of 25. Nurturing a child is like building a pyramid; it's all about laying a solid foundation. Therefore, it is critical to monitor any exposure to screens during these formative years. Finding a balance between life on- and offline is critical. As one very astute occupational therapist, Cris Rowan, says, "The virtual hole is no place to raise a child."[71]

Tips for Creating Balance in a World of Screens

Each child is unique, and some will be more easily drawn to and prefer to spend more time in front of a screen than others. Remember that some people, kids included, may have a predisposition to getting "hooked" on the positive feelings that playing games are designed to provide or the feelings that come with the number of "likes" or "views" on social media postings. Many professionals are now offering some general guidelines to help parents provide a balance and structure for their children's screen usage.

Tip 1. Hold off on getting your child a cell phone as long as possible. In France, beginning in September 2018, cell phones will be banned in schools for children younger than 15. If you have to get your younger child a phone for safety reasons, get a "dumb phone" with limited functions.[72] The goal is to avoid social media/Internet access as long as possible given that middle school students are usually seeking their identity and trying to fit in; also remember that they have pruned those neurons and aren't always making the best decisions. That's why impulsive, unkind, and bullying behaviors can easily occur, creating the perfect storm for misuse of social media.

Tip 2. Limit use of any screens and replace screen time with real time. As one astute mom advises her daughter, "Tether yourself. Tether yourself to real people, conversations, scenery, furry animals, books, music, and the great outdoors. Tether yourself to real life, real people, and real love."[73]

Even the American Academy of Pediatrics (AAP) has expressed concerns about the amount of time that children and teenagers spend with media and about the content they are viewing, and in 2001 the organization recommended the following guidelines: no screen time for ages 0 to 2 years old, one hour a day for 3- to 5-year olds and two hours a day for 6- to 18-year-olds. However, in 2013 the guidelines were revised to reflect more global and less restrictive recommendations. The AAP does acknowledge continued concern about health risks due to excessive screen time and continues to recommend eliminating all screen time for infants aged 0 to 2 years, linking it to language delays. Children and teens should engage with high-quality entertainment media for no more than one or two hours per day. Parents should limit screen time in favor of more brain-building activities, such as those provided in chapter 9.

Questions for pediatricians to incorporate during routine wellness visits to assess patient viewing habits and foster parental education are included in the revised guidelines.[74]

Cris Rowan, a pediatric occupational therapist (OT) and author of *Virtual Child*, and many other OTs would go one step further and recommend no electronic devices until age 12, strictly based on what they know about brain development. Perhaps that is not realistic in today's world, but we strongly encourage you to read articles and books about why you might want to consider limiting these devices for your young children.[75]

Tip 3. Remove all screens from bedrooms and discourage any screen time one to two hours prior to going to bed.

Tip 4. Set "screen-free" times and zones in your home and encourage face-to-face communication instead.

Tip 5. Enable grayscale on phone settings, which will be much less appealing than Technicolor.[76]

Tip 6. Consider getting support from a local professional if you have tried to set limits and boundaries and you get a lot of pushback from your child.

Many therapists and psychologists specialize in screen addictions and can offer advice and a plan for disconnecting from the virtual world, and thus reconnecting with the real world. Dr. Victoria L. Dunckley shares the possible signs to watch for if you suspect that your child may be "hooked" on screens: increased irritability, change in personality and behavior, poor concentration, inability to complete tasks and follow directions, poor grades, low levels of frustration, increased meltdowns, anxiety, stress, feeling overwhelmed, and oppositional behaviors. Before jumping to any conclusions about whether your child has a mental health diagnosis and/or requires medication, she offers the following steps to help parents try an electronic fast for three to four weeks:

1. Parents need to be on the same page and acknowledge that there is a problem with screen usage.

2. Parents need to get all family members and other caregivers onboard and inform the child of the plan to unplug and try some different activities. (Planning and structuring free time is important because that is when screen usage was probably most prevalent.)

3. Parents will need to assess whether there were positive changes and if elimination is the solution or if moderate use of screens is manageable.

Note that it can take several weeks to "reset" and normalize brain function, so be patient. These are hard decisions, and parents may need support during this time, so don't be afraid to ask for professional help.[77] In chapter 9, we offer additional ideas and strategies to help families disconnect from their screens and reconnect to foster relationships and improve communication.

Chapter seven

Achieving Balance in a Busy World

"In order to do what really matters to you, you have to, first of all, know what really matters to you."

—Edward Hallowell, MD

Let us start by saying that there is no perfect life, no perfect parents, no perfect teachers, and no perfect circumstances. As soon as we drop the idea of perfect or ideal, we can start getting real. Letting go of perfection takes the pressure off and allows us to focus on and be present in the life that we have. That being said, we live in a fast-paced, competitive, and overscheduled world that can cause a great deal of stress if we don't learn to find balance.

As much as I know about this topic as a professional, I found myself getting increasingly sucked into an overscheduled world a few years ago. Once my older daughter was well, we were so happy and joyful that we just wanted to partake in everything we could, so we planned one too many trips, and we allowed her to sign up for one too many activities. One day I realized that I had an infant daughter who was not able to have any sort of nap schedule because she was being dragged around to all of her older sister's activities. I was spending half my life in the car and then working very late hours on evenings and weekends to compensate for the lost work time that resulted from managing this incredibly busy schedule. I was burnt out, and we were burnt out as a family! My husband worked all day and then took care of the kids in the evening and much of the weekends when I worked, and I took care of the kids all day and worked evenings and weekends. There was actually very little quality time spent together as a family. Looking back on how we lived for years, it was truly crazy. I became snappy with my children, my husband, and my clients. I felt resentful, and everything felt like work. Then I read a few books on mindfulness and realized that I needed to make some changes, which started by becoming comfortable saying the word "no," and establishing balance and boundaries. This was a process, and it took time, but the rewards were great. Now we put reasonable limitations on what each of us does, and we carve out special time to do something together, just the four of us, each weekend. Once we did this, we all felt better. We are all human. It is easy to get caught up in the rat race, but once we become aware of the detriments of that race, we can choose another, healthier, more fulfilling path.

—*Monica*

Over the past 50 years, the world has changed in many significant ways. Some of those changes include more single parents raising children, more dual-working families, more families on the move (within the United States and abroad), a society that encourages a frenzied pace and heavily rewards winning, and an intrusion of technology and work into our personal time. Some of the consequences of these changes are a loss of routine and traditions, decreased communication within families, seeing others as competitors rather than collaborators, overscheduled calendars, and stressed out children and adults. Let's take a closer look into some of these factors and their impact on parents and children.

Single Parents and Dual-Working Households

We think it probably goes without saying that if one parent has to do the job of two it can result in that parent feeling stressed. Likewise, if both parents have to work long hours outside the home, there may be more stress. The good news is that the workplace seems to be adapting to the changing needs of families. A recent CNN article shared that new technologies and changing family demographics are behind the trend in increased remote work opportunities. Sara Sutton Fell, CEO of FlexJobs, says, "The middle class norm changed from one parent working and one staying at home to two working parents being more common and growth in single-parent families are big factors driving telecommuting to save time when and where you can." The number of work from home jobs has increased by 115 percent since 2005.[1] Many companies are recognizing workers' needs for greater flexibility and are offering flex-time opportunities, such as letting employees set their own eight-hour day, working four longer days to have one weekday off in addition to the weekend, or even cutting back the total number of work hours that constitutes a full-time job.[2]

Transient Families and Workplace Demands

The U.S. Census Bureau reports that the average American moves 12 times during his/her lifetime. The American Moving and Storage Association reports that approximately 83.8 percent of people move within the same state, 13.2 percent move out of state, and 0.33 percent move to another country. Mayflower.com states that 43 million Americans move annually, and the distances they move have increased every year since 1998. Military or government employment–related moves account for about 18 percent of all moves.[3] Sometimes families have to move due to job availability, job transfers, or family situations that require relocation. Moving may increase or decrease time spent with grandparents and other extended family members, which can affect the support and relationships that multigenerational interactions offer.

Another example of a frequent mover or traveler are parents who travel as part of their job responsibilities. As our world and the workplace become more global, more and more jobs are requiring travel. While work travel is often unavoidable, some extra planning for how family time can be protected may make this less stressful for the children.

Blurry Boundaries Between Work and Family Time

It seems like more and more employers have expectations that employees check email, voicemail, and texts in the evening and on weekends. Reporter Daniel Moore addresses this point head-on by saying, "As long as there have been work-issued mobile devices, businesses have turned a blind eye—or an inconsistent one—to a thorny issue underlying the unspoken expectation for employees with those phones and laptops: always be on call." This practice is leading federal regulators to revisit the "de minimus" rule established by the U.S. Department of Labor, which allows employers to disregard what they consider to be "trivial" amounts of work outside the work day. Labor and employment lawyer Darren Weiss says the following of employers and mobile device time, "They expect it, but they don't compensate their employees for it."[4] Though this is only our observation, we see a lot of parents succumb to the pressure to be constantly available to employers. We see more and more parents on the athletic fields, at the park, and at concerts checking and responding to work-related texts or emails or stepping outside to take a work-related call. People feel under pressure to be as available as their coworkers because they fear lack of promotion or even being laid off, which could take away from their ability to provide. Unfortunately, the stress of being constantly available is real. The question becomes how you manage it.

A Fast-Paced and Overscheduled World

Everywhere you look, people are multitasking, their attention is divided, some part of it in the present, while the rest may be thinking of all the things that need to get done later. Work, school, and extracurricular experiences can get busy and overwhelming, and sometimes this sense of organized or unorganized chaos can carry into our home environment. Our homes are supposed to be our safe havens, where we spend time with family and friends, and where we can relax and recharge. But sometimes the scale in our home life can tip in an unhealthy direction. This could look like a lot of physical clutter, stacks and piles, and messes so great it is hard to find things. It could be noise/device clutter, such as a TV on in every room and kids on video games, while Mom or Dad is working on the laptop and trying to get dinner going. It can also look like a whirlwind of appointments and extracurricular activities to shuttle kids to and from with meals frantically wolfed down in between or even on the go. Noisy and chaotic environments can cause children to tune out rather than tune in and can be a source of anxiety and stress. Stress is an important signal from our body that we have crossed some sort of threshold where our body and our brain are thrown out of a state of balance and equilibrium. Stress is our signal that we need to make change. All children and adults need calm and stress-free environments.

Acclaimed psychiatrist and author Edward Hallowell describes this modern life as the "F-state"—frantic, frenzied, forgetful, frustrated, and fragmented—just to name a few.[5] The "F-state" has become such a "way of life" that those who didn't know life before all this craziness wouldn't know there is another way to live.

Rushing children around rarely results in something good. First, when you are under stress, hormones like adrenaline start pumping. Adrenaline is meant to give you a short burst of energy to get through a temporarily stressful situation, but it is not meant to be pumping through your veins all the time. If adrenaline is always pumping, it leads to exhaustion and burnout.

Second, when you are always rushing from point A, to point B, to point C, you rob your kids of the chance to enjoy point A;[6] the focus always becomes moving to the next thing. This devalues the moment and removes focus from what you are currently experiencing. Developing this on-the-go habit also contributes to a mentality in which the process it takes to achieve a result is not as important as the result itself. In an academic context, rather than acknowledging the value of a work ethic, this "rush to the end thought process" gets us focused only on whether the outcome is good or bad (i.e., grade A vs. F). Ultimately, living daily life this way teaches children that life is meant to be fast paced and always moving, and then when they do have the chance to experience downtime they don't see its value or they think it is boring or a "waste of time."

In the documentary *Race to Nowhere*, author Vicki Abeles reveals in great detail the detrimental impact that being overscheduled is having on high school students across America. In her opinion, much of it is driven by the need to build a resume to get into the "right college." Abeles interviews dozens of school administrators who have witnessed the extreme level of stress that high school students are under, and all urge parents to help their children reduce the load.[7]

> *As a counselor who has helped thousands of students with college admissions, I can say that there is a good deal of pressure on students to live busy lives by being successful in athletics, community service, and as leaders of school or community-based clubs, while also being successful academically. After all, they have heard repeatedly in many ways that college admissions counselors are looking for "well-rounded," intelligent applicants. I encourage students and parents to look at the "cost." What is it costing them to maintain their schedule? I have seen more "highly successful" high school juniors and seniors having nervous breakdowns, developing eating disorders, depression and/or anxiety, cutting, using substances to escape, abusing stimulants to stay awake and study later and longer, and developing medical conditions like mono and ulcers. Also, this goal of getting into a prestigious university seems to have diverted many students from understanding the value of the educational process. The focus has been shifted from learning and earning the grade, to getting the grade to get into college. High school teachers will tell you that rather than ask for help kids will often say, "Just tell me what it takes to get an A." It saddens me that there is this somewhat predominant belief system in American society that people only get "somewhere" in life if they attend a highly prestigious school, when there is actually little evidence that attending a highly prestigious or selective college lands graduates in any better of a place in life than attending a non "name brand" school. I like to point out to kids that some of the most successful and wealthy people in society did not attend "name brand" institutions, and in some cases*

they didn't even go to college. The reality is that there are many colleges and universities out there, and it would be nice to see the focus of the admissions process be on finding a great fit for the individual student and not on finding the best "name brand." I would also like students to see and believe that their worth is not determined by a college acceptance letter.

—Monica

Some of the things that result from living in a transient, fast-paced, overscheduled world are:

- Poor mental health: stress, anxiety, and depression
- Poor organization skills: lost materials such as homework, projects, library books, permission forms
- Feeling/experiencing a lack of connectivity with others
- Lack of productivity at school or in the workplace
- Poor or hurried communication
- Loss of free time and family time
- Increase in unhealthy competition

Now let's look a little more deeply at some of the outcomes and solutions to living in this fast-paced overscheduled world.

Changes in Family Routines and Traditions

Frequent moves, the absence of extended family, and the busy world in which we live all affect routines and traditions. The weekly Sunday dinners at Grandmother's house still occur for some families, but certainly not as frequently as they did in the past. It seems hard to get everyone together due to busy schedules of parents and children. There is something to be said about having a leisurely dinner with loved ones. Holiday traditions vary among cultures and families, and some hold strong. Others are being let go, possibly due to time and money factors. Some families maintain routines, whereas others are just getting through the day minute by minute and don't even have time to think about, let alone establish, family routines. Routines and traditions provide structure and predictability for children. This helps them feel safe, secure, and comfortable in knowing what is coming. Anxiety and worries are reduced because their world is predictable, and they feel in control.

One of the most important traditions that is slowly dwindling away is the evening family dinner. Investigators at the University of Minnesota found that traditional family meals have a positive impact on adolescent behavior. In a 2006 survey of nearly 100,000 teenagers across 25 states, the more frequently a family ate dinner together, the more positive values and greater commitment to learning were observed. It is well documented that adolescents from homes having fewer family dinners were more likely to exhibit high-risk behaviors, such as substance abuse, sexual activity, suicide attempts, violence, and academic problems. Dr. Gary Small, professor of psychiatry at UCLA, states, "Actually, it [family dinner] not only strengthens our neural circuitry for human contact, but it also helps ease the stress we experience in our daily lives."[8] Depending on your age, you might remember how dinnertime regularly brought the family together at the end of the day. Parents and children relaxed, shared their day's experiences, kept up with each other's lives, and actually made eye contact while they talked. In today's busy world, some people might consider the traditional family dinner to be unimportant or impossible to make happen on a daily basis. If it does happen, members might tend to eat quickly and return to whatever they were doing prior to dinnertime. As mentioned before, Dr. Small questions whether technology is the cause of the "fractured family." Being working parents ourselves, we believe that there are also other reasons that affect a family's ability to eat dinner together every night. Between work schedules, sports, lessons, and other commitments, sometimes dinner is in the car, at a fast food restaurant, or take out is all that a parent can do. It is now very common to see families out to dinner on school nights, something that rarely happened 50 years ago, and when you do, all of the family members might be on a device while waiting for their meal.

Decreased Communication

> *I remember a college professor telling our class that the norm was 38.5 minutes per week of meaningful conversation between parent and child. That was well over 15 years ago. I suspect due to all the factors addressed in this book that number has decreased.*
>
> *—Perk*

Sometimes communication is in the form of commands, such as "You can eat your breakfast in the car! Hurry up! We're late! Brush your teeth. Get your book bag," rather than give-and-take conversation. We often forget that children need more time to accomplish certain tasks than we do, so sometimes we set ourselves up for failure by not building enough time into the schedule to allow for children to do what they need to do and to have calm conversations.

Communication between parent and child sometimes even comes in the form of texting rather than speaking. It is not unusual for parents and kids in the same house to text one another rather than get up and find one another to talk! This kind of harried communication has led to a decrease in the modeling of a special kind of communication called metacognition (talking aloud about what you are thinking).

I remember a perfect example of "modeling metacognition and problem solving" that happened several years ago when my friend and colleague, Vicki (a school psychologist), was visiting at the shore with her 5-year-old grandson, Dylan. The conversation went something like:

Vicki: "So, what do you think we ought to do today? I just checked the weather. It might rain later this morning. Do you want to go fishing, to the beach, to the boardwalk? What do we want to make sure and do, just in case?"

Dylan: "I want to go fishing."

Vicki: "OK. So what should we do to get ready? Let's see, what do we need?"

Dylan: "My pole. The tackle box. Oh, yeah, bait."

Vicki: "What kind of bait do we need? Chicken? Fish? How about your net? Oh, and we better eat something first. Would you like eggs or cereal?"

Dylan: "Eggs."

Vicki: "Ok, I'll make scrambled eggs. Do you want some toast?"

Dylan: "Yes."

Vicki: "Here is some bread. Perk has wheat and rye. I know you like wheat bread, but I don't think you have ever had rye bread before. Would you like to try it?"

(This conversation allowed for some "voice and choice" and also expanded vocabulary.)

Vicki: "Ok, what do you have to do next?"

Dylan: "Brush my teeth and get dressed."

Vicki: "Yes! Good job. Go ahead and do that, and I'll get ready, too."

This type of nonstop conversation continued during their visit that year. I thought back to previous visits, and it actually started much earlier. I wasn't aware of just what was happening naturally and when there were no time constraints. Trust me when I say it takes time and patience to have these kinds of conversations on a frequent basis, but they are worth it. Vicki was helping Dylan learn language, how to plan ahead, and how to think. He didn't even know it! It was natural for her and became very natural for him, too. Using this as an example, we can all begin to think about modeling conversations with the children we influence.

—*Perk*

Tips for Finding Balance

Tip 1. The first step in making a change is recognition. Decide if your family life feels a little frantic, disconnected, and/or over-scheduled. Consider setting aside time for a family meeting to discuss how everyone is feeling and to determine priorities and a path toward change. Think about holding a regular meeting—maybe one Sunday a month or more or less frequently depending on your family's needs, then you can reevaluate your priorities and progress toward your goals. Staying well as a family requires regular monitoring and check-ins!

Tip 2. Try to establish and stick to routines. Children do best when they know what to expect. Of course life is not always predictable; however, the beauty of a routine is that in times of unpredictability children find comfort in knowing that some things will always stay the same.[9] Having routines helps kids and parents. Try getting everyone involved in picking lunch items and school outfits the night before; this way morning is less frantic. Have an agreed upon homework time each day; this way there is no arguing about when homework gets done.

Tip 3. Foster the spirit of collaboration and working with, not against, others. In an article entitled, "Competing Views on Competition," author Matt Richtel takes a close look at how competition impacts kids. Richtel quotes expert Alfie Kohn as saying, "The evidence overwhelmingly suggests that competition is destructive, particularly, but not exclusively, for kids." However, the article goes on to mention that competition is a part of life, and kids must learn that they aren't always going to be winners. Dr. John Tauer, professor of psychology at the University of St. Thomas, conducted many studies over a five-year period, and the results actually showed that children feel the most satisfaction and give the best performance when they are put in situations that combine cooperation with competition.[10]

Tip 4. Cut back on activities. For example, maybe allow one sport per child instead of two, or allow only one playdate per weekend instead of multiple ones. While children may initially resist these changes, over time, as life feels calmer, they will come to appreciate their new more settled life.

Tip 5. Set aside time to have dinner and conversation with loved ones—whether at your own table or at a restaurant. The research clearly supports the positive effects of sharing a meal as a family. Maybe you can't pull this off every day, but even a few days a week would make a difference! Just remember to disconnect in order to reconnect and leave the mobile devices elsewhere.

Tip 6. Make a point of engaging in in-person/direct communication with family members. Good communication can strengthen family bonds, improve academic performance, help a child learn how to be a good parent someday (learning by example), result in fewer behavior problems and less aggressive behavior, and reduce drug and alcohol abuse.[11] All because parents spend time with and talking with their kids!

Tip 7. Teach your children how to say "No thank you." This of course starts with parents feeling comfortable saying no. Saying no teaches children that we all have to prioritize—none of us are "superheroes," and there are only so many hours in the day. It is healthy to only schedule what you can manage. For the grown-ups, focus on work–life balance where you can. Maybe one parent can get a job that does offer some flexibility around childcare and school needs.

Tip 8. Have a support system. For some people that may be family and extended family, and for others it looks like dinner out with a close group of friends once a month, an annual retreat with long-time friends, or belonging to a church, spiritual group, or volunteer organization. For kids, it may be belonging to a group with common interests like Scouts, a youth group, or a sports team. It is important for kids and for parents to feel connected and supported.

In chapter 9, we offer additional ideas and strategies to help families achieve balance in our overscheduled world.

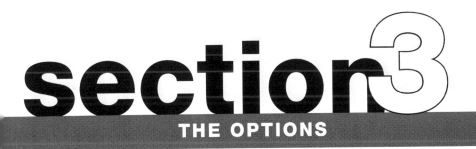

section3
THE OPTIONS

Chapter eight

Parenting Styles

"There are two things we should give our children: one is roots and the other is wings."

—Hodding Carter

"I don't need a manual," said no parent, ever. The reality is that parenting is a hard job that comes with a lot of responsibility, no job description, and no "operator's manual." While parents have managed to raise children for centuries without one, as we discussed in previous chapters, times have changed significantly. As the famous saying goes, "It takes a village," and for a long time, for many people, that village existed. However, today many parents are raising children away from their own families, and often both parents are working full time. Today's parents are facing unprecedented challenges with real concerns regarding food, technology, and changing educational systems, just to name a few. It might offer some reassurance that despite the many changes in society, developmental psychology has shown us that there can be predictable outcomes for children that are largely dependent upon the parenting style employed in the home.

Parenting Styles and Their Outcomes

Research has shown that when a parent picks a distinct style and sticks to it, there are often predictable outcomes for children.[1] Of course, most folks don't sit down one day and decide, "I am going to parent in this style and manner so that my child has this outcome." Instead, most parents end up imitating or avoiding parenting techniques they learned from their own parents and life experiences, by watching child caregivers, and of course the most popular way, through trial and error. Also, it is not uncommon for one parent to have one style and the other parent to have a different style, leading to an overall style that falls somewhere in the middle.

What follows is a basic overview of parenting styles, so that parents can make more informed decisions about their approach to parenting. Like child development, predicting outcomes based on parenting styles is not a perfect science, and there will always be children who break the mold and develop differently than would be expected. We think it is beneficial for parents to understand the four main styles of parenting and their associated outcomes.[2,3]

Authoritarian

Parents who use this approach often believe that children should "be seen and not heard," and that adults are always smarter and always know better. There may not be many conversations about rules or activities in the household because the parent feels it is "my way or the highway" or "because I said so." Many parents who adopt this style tend to be demanding and don't necessarily believe that showing a child warmth or affection is very important. Rather they believe their job is to provide shelter, food, and life's harsh lessons. Fixed rules and beliefs are often enforced, and children are expected to abide by them. Many parents who practice this parenting style do so because that was how they were raised. Typical outcomes for children raised by authoritarian parents:

- Children may have less well-developed communication skills because interactive conversations and debates are not modeled frequently. As a result, children may be less able to negotiate with other children or to consider multiple perspectives.

- Children may take less initiative in their schoolwork and social interactions because they have often been told what to do, and therefore they aren't used to developing their own plan or path. They may also be fearful of making the wrong decisions because they are used to harsh punishments being a consequence.

- Children may have a difficult time considering or understanding beliefs that differ from their own or verbalizing the rationale of their own beliefs because they don't necessarily understand how they were developed.

Many comedy routines have been written over this style of parenting. While it can sometimes be comical to hear adults reflect on the "wooden spoon" or "bars of soap in the mouth" they encountered during childhood, it is important to stop and think about what a physical reaction to anger or frustration teaches children. In their young mind, the lesson learned is: when angry, strike out. If children attempt to manage their anger and frustration on the playground in a physical manner, they are going to find themselves in a lot of trouble. Additionally, research is showing that there can be negative long-term emotional and behavioral consequences for children who have been spanked on a regular basis. The American Psychological Association has taken a strong stand against the use of any physical force in parenting (also referred to as corporal punishment), whether it causes injury or not.[4] Of course, choosing an authoritarian parenting style does not mean that the parent always uses a physical approach to discipline. An authoritarian parenting style may also manifest as one that does not allow for thoughtful discussions between adult and child, wherein the child can practice asking questions and expressing his or her own opinions. Many of the parents we've encountered who employ this style of parenting share that they fear that if they "negotiate" with their children or give them a voice in decision-making, they will no longer be perceived as authority figures. While we certainly agree that parents should be viewed as authority figures, we would also argue that negotiating with children over some decisions does not mean you are handing over control.

Permissive/Indulgent

Parents who use this approach tend to believe that their primary duty as a parent is to make sure their child is happy—and happy at all times. In a permissive household, children tend to end up being in charge, even though the parents may not see it that way. In an attempt to make their children happy, permissive parents often agree to the demands of their children, whether they believe those are the best decisions for their children or not. Rather than consider that children may not know best, the parents will feel that children need to learn how to make their own decisions and then they support or allow them to make those decisions. Parents using this style believe that they are showing their children love by letting them live their lives on their own terms and can usually be swayed to do what the child wants because they don't want to be viewed as "the bad guy." Typical outcomes for children raised by permissive/indulgent parents:

- Similar to children raised in the authoritarian style, these children may have less well-developed social skills because they are used to being appeased and are not used to being challenged by differing opinions or negotiations.

- Children may be less self-assured because they have not been taught to think critically about their own decisions; they just tend to do what feels good in the moment without much regard for the "bigger picture." Furthermore, thinking about the bigger picture may be challenging because they have not developed a good understanding about how to do that or why it is important.

- Children raised in this style may have a good sense of initiative if they are used to making their own decisions or doing things for themselves. However, some children may develop the opposite disposition and become content to sit back and wait for others to do things for them (especially if this is something they become accustomed to their parents doing), thus poor initiative can also be an outcome.

Many parents we've encountered who employ this style of parenting had difficult childhoods themselves. They might share that they were hit for making simple mistakes or were verbally debased for not meeting standards and feel scarred or traumatized by their past experiences. Therefore, their reaction is to be overly responsive and agreeable to their own children's needs. In a sense, these parents let the pendulum swing from one extreme form of parenting to another. We would encourage parents to realize that they are not harming their children by setting reasonable boundaries and predictable and reasonable consequences for behavior.

Authoritative

Many tend to think of this style of parenting as somewhere between Authoritarian and Permissive. Parents who use this method often have high, yet reasonable expectations and standards for their children. They also set firm limits and boundaries about things their children may and may not do and reinforce them with logical consequences. Authoritative parents find a balance between maintaining their role as an authority figure while providing their children with ample and appropriate opportunities to weigh in on decision-making about things that affect them. These parents tend not to believe that they always know what is best for their child. They believe in having discussions with their children and are open to hearing their children's point of view before helping make decisions. While authoritative parents do want their children to be happy, they view their primary duty as a parent to be fostering the development of a self-aware and independent individual.[5,6] Typical outcomes for children raised by authoritative parents:

- Children tend to have well-developed social skills, and they know how to speak for themselves, listen to others, and negotiate.

- Children become more independent over time as the parents' rules and regulations adapt in response to the child's level of maturity.

- Children tend to possess good self-esteem and confidence because they have been encouraged to engage in interactive conversations, which have helped them develop an understanding of their own beliefs/opinions and those of others.

- Children tend to have a high degree of initiative (and even an entrepreneurial spirit) because they have been allowed to try things for themselves and make mistakes. They have learned to understand risks and rewards and how to critically think about things and ask questions without fear of reprimand.

Overall, we find this style of parenting to be a happy medium. It's been our own experience as parents and teachers that when children know what to expect, they feel a greater sense of security that helps them relax and come out of their shell. Also, when children feel like they can approach a parent or a teacher to discuss a problem or issue, they become empowered as they realize they can be an important part of finding solutions.

Uninvolved or Neglectful

Parents who use this style of parenting are often detached from their children. They usually provide for the basic physical needs of the child, but they are not usually found offering guidance and emotional support. They often don't have many rules and regulations because it would take a lot of time or involvement to enforce them. Typical outcomes for children raised by uninvolved/neglectful parents include:

- Children tend to have poorer social and communication skills due to lack of modeling of those skills between parent and child.

- Children may exhibit more behavioral and disciplinary problems in school due to lack of familiarity with structure in the home.

- Children may have increased emotional problems and mental health diagnoses.

- Children may be more susceptible to drugs and/or alcohol abuse in order to escape feelings of sadness or depression.

Researchers have found that oftentimes parents who employ this style of parenting were victims of this style themselves, and they simply did not develop an understanding, from observing their own parents, of all the responsibilities and elements of effective parenting.

Some newer names for parenting styles have made headlines in recent years, such as the "helicopter," "snowplow," or "buddy" parent. When you read the following descriptions, you may recognize a bit of the permissive parenting style in these styles. Parents employing the helicopter style want to fix everything for their children, to prevent them from experiencing any emotional toil or frustration, so they micromanage everything and hover right over top, much the way a helicopter does. Snowplow parents do just that—they plow the way in front of the child and prepare the road for a smooth ride. They might select teachers or coaches and try to set up situations so that their children do not have any bumps along the way. Buddy parents want to be their child's friend, and they don't want to say "no" and become unpopular, so therefore they don't have many rules. Other newly named styles like the "incubator" or "hothouse" parents are concerning. These parents are very concerned with their child's achievements, and they think if they expose them to many forms of tutoring and cognitive stimulation at a young age, they will cultivate children who are more intelligent and successful.[7] However, as we shared in the brain and child development chapters, by and large, brain development cannot be rushed. Therefore, this style of parenting may cause a child to feel a lot of pressure, and ultimately backfire, potentially leading to mental and physical health woes rather than greater achievement. These parenting styles have only recently been identified, and there is not enough long-term research to determine if they lead to specific and predictable outcomes for child behavior.

The styles of parenting that were shared earlier in this chapter (authoritarian, permissive, authoritative, and neglectful) were named and categorized by developmental psychologists many years ago, so the terms may not sound overly familiar to all readers. However, they have been extensively studied over long periods of time, and there is some practical advice based on the outcomes. By and large, the parenting style that has the best overall outcomes for kids is the authoritative style.

A Case for Authoritative Parenting

Children raised by parents utilizing an authoritative style tend to take initiative because they have been given responsibility and the opportunity to try different tasks and experiences and to make mistakes without swift punishment. They also tend to have better communication and negotiation skills because they have been actively involved in conversations and decision-making. In order to make it in college or the job market, one has to take initiative and responsibility and be a good communicator, so it seems to us that this is a good model to emulate. What actions can you take to employ an authoritative style?

- Have conversations with your children. Ask them how they feel about different things that happen in their world. Listen as much as you talk.

- Process the results of their choices. When they make good choices, reflect on the choice made and why the outcome was good. When the outcome was poor, discuss alternative choices that might have led to a better outcome.

- Have rules that are fair. Discuss why the rules are in place and allow for some questions and answers regarding those rules. If children understand why the rules exist, then they are more likely to respect them.

- Be consistent in enforcing the rules. While of course there are special occasions for cutting some slack or making an exception, by and large, if you consistently enforce rules, they become predictable and respected.

- Talk about feelings. When something upsets you, makes you angry, or makes you feel really happy or proud, stop in that moment and say, "When you do this, I feel X." Let your children know that they should do the same in turn. Doing so helps children learn how to communicate about feelings.

- Model good conflict resolution skills. If you are too angry to have a fair or reasonable discussion, tell your children you need to cool down. Likewise, afford them the same opportunity if they seem too stressed to have a good discussion.

In learning about parenting styles, we have the opportunity to understand that oftentimes specific and direct actions will have specific and direct consequences. Now we can be active participants in choosing a parenting style. If you recognize that your parenting style fits into one of the categories above, and you feel like you may already be off on the "wrong foot," there is always the opportunity to make a change. You can talk to your children and tell them you feel that you want to try something new. Explain that just like them, you are not perfect, and that sometimes, as adults, we learn important life lessons, and that it is never too late to change, grow, or learn!

Parents' Role in Character Development

Our experience has shown us that kids who possess certain key personality characteristics tend to fare better in the classroom, during unstructured time (like on the playground), and eventually upon entry to college or the workforce. Parents have a powerful opportunity to instill character education in their households, and in this section we introduce and explain some of those key characteristics.

Empathy

Empathy is being sensitive to and aware of the feelings and thoughts of others. In other words, being able to put yourself in someone else's shoes. However, the bad news is that teens today are 40 percent less empathetic than those of 30 years ago.[8] In her book, *UnSelfie: Why Empathetic Kids Succeed in Our All-About-Me World*, Michelle Borba, explains that "empathy is the one human capacity that allows us to link minds and hearts across cultures and generations to transform our lives.[9] Children are wired for goodness, but culture and parenting can help or hinder their potential to become empathetic leaders and change makers."[10] The good news is that parents and educators can easily change that statistic by "raising our children from the inside out." We must model, teach, and expect empathy from all children.

Resilience and Grit

Resilience is the ability to recover from or adjust to life's challenges.[11] Grit is having unyielding courage in the face of hardship.[12] Resilience and grit often go hand in hand, and are not fixed traits that you're either born with or not. Resilience and grit develop as people grow and gain life experiences that equip them with more knowledge about the world and themselves, and enables them to be better at thinking critically and self-management. These traits also come from healthy and supportive relationships with parents, peers, and others, as well as cultural beliefs and traditions that help people cope with the inevitable bumps in life. Again, like empathy, parents can help their children develop resilience and grit. It takes courage not to overprotect and shelter your children, as it can be uncomfortable to see them upset or frustrated. However, resisting the urge to swoop in and "save" them from being disappointed, unhappy, or frustrated is exactly what will allow them to develop resilience and grit.

Be assured that there are things that parents can do that will nurture resilience and grit. Dr. Kenneth Ginsburg, a pediatrician who specializes in adolescent medicine at Children's Hospital of Philadelphia, says "resilience is about bouncing back. However, the challenge is to prepare kids to have the capacity to recover before anything actually goes wrong."[13] He shares "7 Cs" as important traits that help build resilience. [14]

Competence describes the feeling of knowing that you can handle a situation well. Encourage competence by allowing your child to help with making decisions.

Confidence develops as a child begins to believe in his or her own abilities. Assist in building confidence by providing specific praise about effort rather than outcome.

Connections can be built with family, friends, and community. Foster connections by allowing the expression of emotions and discussing conflict openly to resolve problems. Close ties with others will instill a sense of security and prevent children from seeking destructive alternatives to love and attention.

Contributions to the world help our children recognize that the world is a better place because they are in it. Try providing opportunities for your children to contribute in your home and community by doing chores or reaching out to help others.

Coping effectively with stress will help your children be better prepared to overcome life's challenges. It may be helpful to brainstorm and model positive and effective coping strategies on a consistent basis.

Control of outcomes of their decisions will help children feel empowered and more resilient in various situations. Allow your children to have "voice and choice" in structured settings. Help them understand that they can always make a positive choice in any situation.

Character building develops a solid set of morals and values. Help build character by having ongoing discussions about how behaviors affect others. Every day there are "teachable moments" that can nurture and foster development of good character.

In recent years there has been some interesting commentary by college coaches in the media about youth and character. Tom Izzo, Michigan State University men's basketball team coach, is somewhat of a legend. When recruiting, he states, "I look for a well-rounded person. I figure anyone who is potentially playing at this level is pretty driven as an athlete. I want to see if they have people skills, if they are a multidimensional person. Most important, I want to see evidence of a good character." So how does he do this? He gets one home visit and that's it. He says,

> I look at how that young man treats his parents. Is he respectful? Is he polite? Does he use manners toward them as well as toward me? You can tell if the way a son treats his mother is genuine—there's no faking that

relationship. I know if a son is respectful to his parents, he's been taught to respect his coach.

So, what is Coach Izzo's inside advice to raising a champion athlete? "Don't try. Instead, instill in children the character of a champion and watch how far they'll go."[15]

Bullying and Conflict Resolution

A challenging situation that many children will encounter during their school experience is bullying. The term "bully" or "bullying" is likely familiar to most of us and is a word that carries strong connotations. Because bullying is something many parents will have to help their child with, it is important to understand what bullying means and to use the term in appropriate ways. Bullying is aggressive behavior that involves negative actions, is repeated over a period of time, and involves an imbalance of power or strength. There are three types of bullying: verbal (saying or writing mean things, including cyberbullying), social (hurting someone's reputation or relationships), and physical bullying. That being said, a one-time incident, such as a child being cornered by another child and physically hurt or threatened, can be serious and would require swift adult intervention.

Many times, children and parents use the word bullying to describe an upsetting, though relatively harmless, incident that happened on the playground, bus, or in the neighborhood. As children engage in social situations, they will naturally "try on" different behaviors, and they will make mistakes. Most young children are not deliberately mean, and one unkind comment or action does not constitute bullying. However, it's important to address unkind behaviors and teach kindness, empathy, positive social interactions, and how to resolve conflicts peacefully. Many times, the source of a conflict is a misperception of a situation. Misunderstandings and lack of coping skills can cause frustration, confusion, sadness, and anger. These feelings may lead some children to the conclusion that they are being bullied, a term that they hear frequently. Therefore,

it is important to understand whether your child is truly being bullied. Many schools have programs designed to help children and
parents understand what constitutes bullying, the roles we all play
(bully, victim/target, bystanders, and upstanders—those who come
to the aid of the victim and stand up to the bully), and how to
respond.[16] In the event that ongoing discussions with your child
lead you to believe that the behavior in question could indeed be
considered bullying behavior, it's important to recognize, acknowledge, and take steps to prevent it from reoccurring.

Depending on the severity of what your child is encountering,
you may need to request a meeting with school personnel, such as
the classroom teacher, school counselor, and/or principal. Together
you can develop a plan to address the bullying. We would also like
to mention that if you are worried that your child is the bully, you
can still reach out to school staff to develop an action plan to work
through the concerning behaviors.

Showing your child that reaching out for help is a sign of
strength, not weakness, is an important role-modeling opportunity
in and of itself. However, in your own home, you can also teach,
model, practice, and reinforce conflict resolution skills. If your
child shares a situation in which he or she felt hurt or upset, it is
important to help your child process the event, whether you feel the
event was a big deal or not. Parent and child can brainstorm ideas
for solving the problem. Here are some ideas to try:

- Work through various "what if" scenarios. For example,
  "What would you say if that happened again? I'll play Johnny,
  and you be you. Tell me what Johnny did, so I can say/do
  just what Johnny did." You start, and then let your child finish. Listen carefully to what is said, and then in return you
  can say, "If someone said that to me, I would feel X." Then
  offer the reason why. By talking things through you offer
  your child insight into how someone else might be feeling or
  misunderstanding the exact same scenario.

- Use feeling words on a regular basis, such as happy, sad, angry, frustrated, and so forth. Having the right words to explain feelings leads to better communication.

- Talk to your child about how people send signals in ways other than words. You could look through a magazine and collect some pictures of different facial expressions and show them to your child. You could say, "How do you think that person is feeling?" If your child seems to be reading the expressions, that's great, but if not, you could point out, "Do you see how her face looks bright red and her fists are clenched? To me that looks like she is getting angry." Or, "Do you see how his eyes are facing downward and he has a little bit of a frown? I think he seems sad."

- Talk about different scenarios that could occur on the playground, classroom, or other social situations and help your child decide which times might be best to reach out to an adult for help versus first trying to solve the problem independently. If your child runs for help every single time there is an issue, other children may perceive him or her as a "tattle-tale," which could make establishing friendships more difficult.

- If your child is in daycare, preschool, or elementary age, you could also ask the caregiver or teacher for feedback about how your child is resolving conflicts. This way you can get some idea of how much work you may or may not need to do to enhance this skill.

Taking this approach offers children options and strategies to resolve an ongoing situation or other challenging situations they may face in the future.

As children develop coping and conflict resolution skills, they become empowered and feel more confident and competent. They learn to overcome problems and "bounce back" from challenging situations or disappointments. They develop "grit" and resilience.

What may be more challenging is for parents to sit back and give their children a little room to feel challenged and unsettled by difficulty. As parents we often want to fix things or make them better, and sometimes we jump in too soon.[17] We hope that when parents have a better understanding of how working through challenges empowers children, they will feel more comfortable observing struggles and only stepping in when absolutely necessary.

Our job as parents is to raise our children to leave the nest. They have to find their way in this world because we won't always be there for them. What better gift to give a child than a strong personal character and a toolbox of coping skills!

Chapter nine

Strategies That Build a Strong Foundation

"It's not what you do for your children, but what you have taught them to do for themselves, that will make them successful human beings."

—Ann Landers, writer and advisor

While we may not be able to control the environment outside our own homes, we can make some purposeful decisions about the way we raise and interact with children to help them reach their full potential.

Raising Kids from the Ground Up

A strong foundation is critical to building a structure that will withstand environmental assault and the test of time.

We feel the same can be said for raising children and have constructed a pyramid to serve as a visual model for raising a child who will thrive in today's world (figure 9.1). The pinnacle of the pyramid is a thriving human being, but how do you get there? By having sturdy steps to climb!

You can see how the foundation of this pyramid starts with you, the parent. The building blocks that lay the foundation are ones you must provide in your own home. As your child grows, more people step in and help solidify additional blocks by building or strengthening important skills. That's where the "village" comes in. These people might include family members, neighbors, friends, educators, doctors, coaches, scout leaders, spiritual/religious leaders, or anyone else who takes an interest in your child's well-being and development. The village is large, but without it, a parent's job can be more difficult.

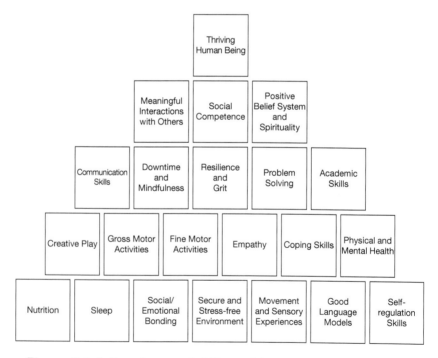

Figure 9.1 A Developmental Pyramid

Using the steps of the pyramid as a guide, the following strategies and suggestions are what we've observed and confirmed in our own lives to be the most critical, practical, and affordable ways to have an impact on your child's brain and body development.

Nutrition

Just like a car needs gas, our bodies need fuel. Food has changed, and today's Standard American Diet (SAD) does not always help to build healthy bodies and brains. Many of the foods that kids consume may not provide adequate vitamins, minerals, and nutrients, and, at times, they may contain substances that aren't healthy. Good nutrition can increase energy levels, concentration, performance, and moods. For more information about nutrition, see chapter 4.

- Purchase fresh, healthy and organic foods whenever possible. When budget is an issue, avoid foods on the "Dirty Dozen" list and prioritize buying those on the "Clean 15" list.

- Limit the amount of carbohydrate-rich foods such as breads, crackers, chips, pretzels, and any other processed foods. Avoid the "ites" and "ates" (i.e., nitrites, nitrates, sulfites, sulfates).

- Avoid foods that are marked "light" or "fat free," as they often use artificial sweeteners to reduce the caloric intake. Full-fat dairy products are now considered to be acceptable, and often recommended, especially for young children with developing brains.

- Remember to consume five key brain nutrients every day: protein, vitamins, minerals, natural fats and oils, and water.

- Many children need to eat every two hours in order to keep their blood sugar levels stable.

- For those looking for potential food interventions for ADD/ADHD, try removing gluten and dairy products from the diet.

Normally these foods have to be out of the diet for three to four straight weeks before any significant improvement may be noted.

- Be aware of the signs of nutrient deficiencies and talk to your doctor or nutritionist. Many children do have deficiencies. We tell parents if it looks like a duck and quacks like a duck, it's probably a duck, so if you are concerned, be persistent and firm about what you are noticing or experiencing when talking to your doctor.

Sleep

Everyone needs sleep; however, it is especially important for children's mental and physical development. In fact, children will spend 40 percent of their childhood asleep! Sometimes, what looks like cranky and oppositional behavior could be a case of just being overtired. Children need their sleep, including naps when younger, and appropriate bedtimes at all times.[1] Consider the following as a guideline for the amount of sleep people need based on age:[2]

- 2 to 5 years: 10 to 13 hours/night (may include an afternoon nap for the younger ones)

- 6 to 13 years: 9 to 11 hours/night

- 14 to 17 years: 8 to 10 hours/night

- Adults: 7 to 9 hours/night

If your child isn't getting enough sleep or is having trouble falling asleep, you can try the following tips:

- Consider no screens in bedrooms, especially in children's rooms, as the electromagnetic radiation they emit may affect sleep.[3]

- No screen usage one to two hours prior to bedtime; read paper books instead. This will allow the brain to quiet and get ready for a good night's sleep.

- Serve a light protein-rich snack 30 minutes before your child lies down to sleep. A full tummy allows for more stable blood sugar levels and a better night's sleep. For some children, it prevents waking up "hangry" (hungry-angry). Avoid caffeine in the afternoon and evening.

- Have a bedtime routine that is predictable and consistent. This will help to avoid bedtime struggles because it's just "what we do" every night. Predictable routines help your child feel secure and comfortable and less likely to balk at bedtime.

Social and Emotional Bonding

Social-emotional development refers to a child's self-confidence, trust, empathy, and competencies in language usage and cognitive curiosity. Strong social-emotional development is a predictor of later academic, social, and emotional success.[4] In order to foster healthy social and emotional bonding, a close relationship with one or both parents is critical, especially during the first two years. Children who experience this type of bonding are less likely to exhibit negative emotional behaviors during later years.

- Cuddle under a blanket and tell stories or read books.

- Listen and dance to music together.

- Disconnect to reconnect with your children by cutting back on screen time. Consider turning off the TV and other devices during mealtimes, playtime, bath time, and bedtime.

- Leave special messages in your child's lunch bag, in his or her desk at school, or in his or her assignment book.

- Consider coming up with new traditions that can help slow down the pace of life—let your children be involved in this process! These can include special holiday traditions or more routine things that your family does. They might include: Friday pizza and movie night, a special family birthday tradition, going out for ice cream on the last day of school, or whatever else your family values and enjoys.

- Tell your child "I love you" often and unconditionally.

Secure and Stress-Free Environment

Stress is normal and, in many ways, can be helpful for maintaining attention, motivating us to complete tasks, and even develop feelings of competence and resilience. So, stress can actually be a good thing.[5] This type of good stress is called eustress and can be the impetus to get that project done by the deadline or the feelings you have when you are getting ready for that dream vacation. Short-term stress can cause elevated levels of cortisol that are normal; in fact, many people have higher levels of cortisol in the morning to give them energy to navigate their day.

However, distress is negative stress. It can prevent us from getting things accomplished, and when it is chronic, it can cause the body to release too much cortisol, a chemical hormone that is released to manage stress. Too much chronic stress can cause heart disease, a rise in blood pressure, a weakened immune system, and can contribute to diabetes and cancer.[6] While our lives will never be stress-free, we can adjust the way we respond to stress. Children need to feel safe and secure in a "distress-free" environment.

- Consider establishing routines for the morning, coming home from school, homework, and bedtime. When children know what to expect, it helps them feel secure and decreases stress and anxiety, because things are predictable. They don't have to worry and wonder about what is happening next or "what if" scenarios. The more children experience family routines, the more independent they become, which builds feelings of competence and confidence. For young children, consider making a checklist to help them remember the daily routines. This can be as simple as a sticky note, or if they are too young to read, draw simple pictures to represent the tasks.

- Create structure and organizational systems to make your life easier. Try to keep up with materials management in order to reduce clutter and keep up with organizational tasks. An acronym that often helps is OHIO (only handle it once). For example, check the homework folder, sign the field trip permission form right away, put it back in the folder, and be done.

- Make a daily checklist for yourself to help you stay organized.

- Consider the tips we offer in chapter 7 for combating an overscheduled, busy life!

Movement and Sensory Experiences

Children learn through movement and hands-on experiences. According to Harvard psychiatrist and author Dr. John Ratey, exercise and movement actually build brain cells.[7] As we discussed in chapter 5, this is the reason that play is so important for the developing brain and body. Exploring the world by using the five senses enhances learning and makes it memorable and fun.

It's important to get children up and moving frequently. Children are not small adults; their nervous and sensory systems are still developing and need more stimulation than adults. A good rule of thumb is to expect them to be able to focus on a single assigned task for the same number of minutes as their age. For example, a 7-year-old may only be able to focus for seven minutes, especially on a nonpreferred task or challenging task. Having said that, a small group of young children who are actively engaged in an interesting task might be able to remain on-task for 15 to 30 minutes, but then they will need a movement opportunity.[8] Some activities you could do with your child are:

- Explore nature and go for hikes/walks. Spending time in green, outdoor settings nurtures happiness and a state of calm and is definitely important for brain and body development (see chapter 5 for more on this).

- Grow a garden or "pick your own" produce at local orchards or community gardens during the growing season.

- Visit "Please Touch" museums and exhibits that allow active participation; these are perfect for developing bodies and brains/minds.

- Make a "sensory table" at home

Many preschool and elementary classrooms have sensory tables. To make one at home, fill a container with sand, rice, gravel, seeds, etc. and bury small items. Have your child dig down deep to discover the buried surprises. Ideas are plentiful on Pinterest and other online resources. Just search on "sensory bins" or "sensory activities."

For children who are more sensitive to sensory experiences (sensory defensive), consider that clothing can affect their experience or mood (i.e., tight vs. loose fits, soft vs. rough textures, scratchy tags or seams). If your child expresses discomfort, simply changing clothing could positively impact his or her overall sense of comfort and security. The same applies to the experience of physical contact with others. For example, a sensitive child may perceive touch from another person as more aggressive and hurtful than it was intended.

Some children actually need more sensory input (sensory seeking) and respond well to wearing a weighted vest or holding a weighted stuffed animal in their lap. These self-regulating tools provide proprioceptive input and deep pressure that can be calming and help focus the nervous systems. In addition, the extra sensory feedback from the weight can reduce anxiety and also help with insomnia.

Lastly, if extra stimulation is needed, consider getting a fidget item for your child. Fidget items like a squishy ball, springy cord, or kneadable erasers can keep hands busy and provide sensory input, which can sometimes improve listening skills and reduce anxiety. Rubber bands around the two front desk legs can be a good outlet for fidgety feet.

Good Language Models

Children learn language from their parents or caretakers. Providing a rich language environment by increasing the number of vocabulary words that children hear and know and speaking clearly are critical skills to future language and academic success.[9] When children don't hear sounds and words pronounced clearly and correctly, this can have a negative effect on receptive and expressive language development, phonological awareness skills, reading, spelling skill development, and written expression. Many learning delays or disabilities are rooted in language delays. Read to/with your children as early and often as you can. Language shapes so many parts of life (culture, thinking, the brain itself, etc.), so it is important to talk with your kids—even before they can talk back! Tell stories, read nursery rhymes, sing songs, have conversations, and play simple word games like:

- "I Spy something that is very large, brown and black, has two ears . . . (the family dog)." Use attributes/adjectives to develop language, such as, "I see something under the table," "on top of the shelf," or "next to the refrigerator."

- "I'm going on a picnic/trip and I'm going to take an apple . . .": the next person repeats the sentence and adds something that begins with b, the third person repeats the sentence with both items and adds a third beginning with c, and so on.

- "I'm thinking of something that is a tool (category), used to hang pictures (function), has a cylinder shaped wooden handle and a metal top with a claw on one end and a round pounding part on the other (attributes)." "Is it a hammer?" your child asks. Understanding categories, functions, and attributes are key ingredients to language development.

Self-Regulation Skills

Self-regulation is a child's ability to do and to not do. It is the new fourth R of school (reading, 'riting, 'rithmetic, and regulate).[10] The abilities to self-regulate and delay gratification are strong predictors for future academic success, happiness, and good health, and even increases potential earning power later in life! Therefore, it is critical that children are taught to regulate their behavior for the situation at hand. Children need a parent's guidance to learn that there are acceptable behaviors for different times and places. They need to be aware of their surroundings and act accordingly, which often means that they have to regulate their bodies and behavior.

Children need opportunities to practice patience. They may need some coaching to get through certain experiences, such as exercising patience before interrupting speaking adults to ask for something while sitting in church or waiting their turn. It is okay to say something like, "I promise you will be okay waiting for a couple minutes." Some children may have a small meltdown while waiting, and this is okay because afterwards they will realize that they are actually okay even though they did not receive immediate gratification. This may also be a good time to teach them the difference between a "real" reason to interrupt (i.e., baby brother knocked over the candle and the dining room tablecloth is on fire) versus one that is not urgent (i.e., I want you to help me find my toy).

- Delaying gratification is a very important, lifelong skill. Consider having your children save for a "big ticket" item. For allowance earnings or when children receive money as a gift, consider giving a portion to charity or putting a portion in long-term savings. Then the remainder can be for spending.

- Help your children learn to become more aware of how their body's ability to regulate is working. Is it too slow, too fast, or, just right? You can use common visuals to help younger children reflect and evaluate their behavior. For example, use a "putt-putt" car (old fashioned car) to represent sluggish and slow behavior. A fancy Corvette or "souped-up" car could represent behavior that is too fast or hyped up, and another regular car could represent "just right" behavior.[11]

- Be consistent; say what you mean and mean what you say. Children need, but will often resist, discipline. Children are better able to learn to respect discipline when it is consistent and predictable. Their behavior is often their way of asking for limits and boundaries, and it's up to parents to establish them.

Creative Play

Creative, imaginative play is a critical component to healthy brain and body development. Play provides a strong foundation for intellectual growth, creativity, and problem solving. It also helps nurture emotional and social skills development. In the twenty-first century, creative problem solvers, independent thinkers, and people with strong social skills will be more successful than those who do not possess those skills.[12] Children who engage in play develop many other skills, including language, self-regulation, and gross and fine motor skills. Play can also reduce anxiety and depression. Rough-and-tumble play actually develops executive function skills and may help children with ADD/ADHD control their impulsivity and concentrate in school. For more information on the benefits of play, see chapter 5.

- Encourage your child to go outside and play whenever possible.
- Simplify your environment. Fewer toys will benefit children in the long term as they will have to develop their creativity and find other brain-nurturing activities to do. In a recent article, author, Joshua Becker, states, "I'm not anti-toy. I'm just pro-child. So, do your child a favor today and limit the number of toys." Some of the pros of having fewer toys include:[13]

  ○ Increased creativity, perseverance, and attention spans

- Learning to take greater care of things (because there aren't many backup options)

- Developing a greater love of reading, writing, art, and music, as you can participate in these without toys

- Less arguing and selfishness

- Living in a less cluttered environment

• When purchasing toys for your children, ask yourself, "Will this toy have more than one purpose, and will it nurture my child's imagination?"

Gross Motor Activities

Gross motor skills include large movements of the body like running, jumping, skipping, and climbing and are critical for strengthening bones and muscles and developing core strength (abdominal). Strong core strength helps with stamina, posture, and sitting upright for future school tasks, including writing. Before children can engage in more complex gross motor activities that combine many movements like what would be needed to navigate the soccer field or execute a routine in gymnastics, they need time to focus on individual skills. A child with weak gross motor skills may feel uncoordinated and in-competent in physical activities, such as neighborhood or playground games, and this can sometimes affect peer relationships. Developing these skills means that your child is on the go and getting exercise, and exercise and movement builds brain cells.[14] If you can get your children hooked on physical activity as a child, this may lead to a more active and healthier adult, which is critical as one ages.[15]

One thing you can do is allow opportunities for fun and help-ful "heavy work" because heavy work engages muscles and builds muscle tone. These activities can improve attention, alertness level (too slow, too fast, or just right), body awareness, and muscle tone and can also decrease sensory defensiveness.[16] These may include activities like:

- Whole-body actions such as carrying things (groceries, laundry), pushing or pulling objects (vacuum, broom, mop, wagon full of things, shopping cart), running, climbing, jumping, tugging (tug-of-war), digging in the garden, or building a fort with pillows and blankets.[17]

- Oral actions like chewing, sucking, and blowing (bubbles).

- Use of hands for squeezing (cookie dough, play dough, toothpaste tube), pinching (clothespins, clay, toys like Lite Brite or Legos), or "fidgeting."

Other things you can do include encouraging your child to engage in sensory play to enhance learning by whole-body and three-dimensional exploration; building in trips to the local playground where children can engage their large muscle groups by climbing ladders, hanging from the monkey bars, and pumping their legs on the swings; buying or constructing a tunnel—tunnels force kids to crawl well beyond when the crawling stage is done, and crawling engages core muscles and the building of connections between the left and right brain; and/or enrolling your child into a class that involves movement for at your local gym or YMCA. Learning to swim is another great activity, and it's important in order to keep kids safe. Movement in water strengthens muscles more rapidly than playing on the floor because the resistance while swimming in water activates more large-muscle groups. It causes the brain to develop through bilateral, cross-patterning movements, which just means crossing the midline and getting the right and left brains working together. Research shows that getting kids swimming early on improves physical, mental, emotional, and cognitive development and increases self-confidence.[18]

Fine Motor Activities

Fine motor skills involve the use of the little muscles in our body like fingers, toes, wrists, lips, and tongue and are critical for completing tasks like eating with utensils, cutting with scissors, zipping jackets, tying shoelaces, buttoning buttons, opening jars, and writing. Many children are starting school with poor habits due to weak hand muscles. These habits are hard to change and can result in children holding their pencil with a maladaptive grip, which makes writing laborious and illegible.[19] The good news is there are many things parents can do to strengthen these muscles, as well as improve overall coordination and hand-eye coordination. The secret is to encourage these activities early on and make the activities fun and engaging![20]

We encourage parents to use the preschool years to develop hand strength by engaging in fun, multisensory activities. Years ago, young children were provided fat crayons and pencils, with the thinking being "bigger is better" for little hands. This is actually not true. Bigger, thicker markers, pencils, and crayons are actually more difficult for young children. Their writing utensils need to be scaled to the size of their hands, and that means "smaller is better." Provide small pieces of chalk or crayons to naturally establish the proper "tripod grip" so necessary for handwriting. When a crayon is broken in half, it becomes so small that it actually forces the child to use a proper tripod grasp. A golf pencil is another option. There are also "pipsqueak" markers and "rock crayons" for little hands (see appendix). The smaller, the better for establishing an effective pencil grip. The following are some more ways that you can help develop your child's fine motor skills:

- Mount a chalkboard on the wall or place a large paper on an easel for upright writing (standing while writing on a wall or easel). Then offer small utensils for writing or small pieces of sponges with some paint for sponge painting. Q-tips for painting also make for a fun activity. This will stimulate a proper grip without your children even knowing.

- Provide a variety of hands-on activities like arts and crafts, puzzles, shape games, building blocks, and playdough. These are all good for developing spatial skills that often are linked to success in fields like science, technology, engineering, and math.

- Help in the kitchen by kneading dough or stirring batter. Using cookie cutters on rolled out dough gives a good fine motor workout.

- Provide playtime with water or sand and a variety of containers. Most children never tire of playing in sand or spending extra time in the bathtub or a little pool in the summer, and these experiences cost very little money. Children can learn about math and science concepts like the properties of liquids and solids, whether objects will sink or float, and the concepts of density, weight, and volume, all of which are easily explored with sand and water.[21]

- Find ways to play with "chip clips" or "clothespins"—the squeezing motion used to pinch the clip open develops the muscles needed for proper pencil grip. Encourage pinching the clip with the thumb underneath and pointer and middle fingers on top, rather than using the whole hand.

- Use little rubber stamps and ink to make pictures or cut sponges into small pieces and dip in paint to create designs or sponge paintings.

- String pasta, Cheerios, or Fruit Loops on string or yarn to make a necklace or bracelet.

- Tear little pieces of construction paper or tissue paper using the thumb, pointer, and middle fingers to make the tear. Then roll the piece up in a ball and make a "mosaic" type of picture by gluing the little pieces on paper.

- Teach your child how to tie shoelaces. This takes patience and lots of practice but is a skill that most children can master by 6 or 7 years of age. To start, try tying a bathrobe tie, as it is typically thicker and easier for small hands to manage. Allow it to hang in front of the child, perhaps on a doorknob. It's sometimes easier to start learning to tie when facing the task head on, literally. Then you can try putting it around the child's waist and teach tying while looking down. When moving to shoelaces, start with two thick laces that are different colors before attempting tying with two skinny, single color laces. There are several ways to approach this, and tips can be found in the appendix.

Empathy

Empathy is the ability to feel what other people might be feeling. It's the ability to "put one's self in another's shoes." "Identifying, understanding, and expressing emotions are the skills kids need to activate empathy," says Michele Borba, author of *UnSelfie: Why Empathetic Kids Succeed in Our All-About-Me World*. Many researchers and educators, including Borba, would say there is an increase in peer cruelty and that empathy is one skill that is lacking in today's youth, with teens now 40 percent lower in empathy levels than 30 years ago.[22] Why? Many studies indicate that the increased amount of time kids are spending behind screens and our high-pressure culture are partly to blame. Being behind a screen doesn't allow one to see the reactions of another person, so it's easier to say or do an unkind thing. It's up to parents to teach children to be empathetic, and the good news is that it can be done.

- Teach your children feeling words like happy, sad, angry, afraid, surprised, disgusted, frustrated, and proud; many others can be added as your child develops.

- Read to and with your child early on and don't stop just because they can read. Consider a variety of book genres that foster discussion about empathy. For example, the book *Have You Filled a Bucket Today?* by Carol McCloud uses the metaphor of filling a bucket to represent doing good deeds for others, or doing something kind. Be sure to catch your child being "a bucket filler," and praise him or her for doing that. You will see the smile grow from ear to ear!

- There is always time for a good movie night with family and friends. Consider "movies with a message." There are many movies that foster meaningful family discussions and provide opportunities to teach empathy and other valuable life lessons to your children. Following the movie, ask some simple questions: "How did you feel when you saw that?" "How do you think character X was feeling?"

- Help your child see others' perspectives. Observe your child playing or interacting with others, then later say something like, "Do you think you did a good job of sharing/letting Johnny take a turn?" Also offer positive feedback, "It was nice to see you listen to Johnny's story without interrupting."

- Spend time with or doing things for those less fortunate via church or community outreach programs. Many children don't understand how fortunate they are until they see others who are less fortunate.

- Model and include your child in doing random acts of kindness. You might ask periodically, "What did you do that was kind today?" "Did you see anyone else being kind today? How?"

Coping Skills

Learning to cope when things don't go our way or when we are faced with adversity, distress, or challenges is a critical life skill. Without coping skills, children can become easily overwhelmed and may rely on others to help them through tough times. The following are ways you can help foster coping skills in your child:

- Help your children become aware of the physical signs of frustration, anger, sadness, or any significant change in their emotional state (hands in fists, lips pursed, face is red, feet are tapping, etc.) or hear their inner voice before a meltdown occurs. You can prompt with, "I can tell you are getting frustrated/angry/sad because I see your face turning red. When I feel that way, I take a few deep breaths and take a break."

- Have your child practice deep breathing; this is always a good strategy for everyone to use and is the fastest way to reduce stress. Breathe in for two counts, hold for three counts, breathe out four counts, and then start again (call it 2-3-4 breathing). Some counselors of young children will say, "Take a deep breath, hold it, and now blow out your worries," or they may have the child write down worries on a piece of paper and then put it through a shredder or tear it up and throw the worries away. Yoga instructors often suggest repeating this mantra to yourself or in a soft voice, "I am breathing in, and I am breathing out." Take a deep breath in, hold, and then slowly release. This can also help one fall asleep.

- Teach your child how to tolerate discomfort and uncertainty. You can say something like, "I know this feels really hard, and that's okay. Sometimes we learn the most when we feel challenged."

- Model your use of coping skills when faced with adversity. Teach and provide guided practice of coping strategies (stay calm, count to 10, deep breaths, walk away, etc.).

- Help your children distinguish between perceived and real causes for worry or anger. You might even help them quantify the level of worry/anger by using a numeric rating scale or attaching words/visuals for degree of emotion. For example, an anger/worry thermometer might start with a picture of a breezy, sunny day. Then it might continue with a storm cloud and increased winds and eventually end up in a tornado/hurricane state.

- Model and practice self-talk during frustrating situations. Sometimes saying something simple like, "That was hard for me too when I was your age," helps them to feel connected to your sense of empathy for them.

- Give your children opportunities to practice "what if" scenarios. This "mental rehearsal," as it is sometimes called, can help them feel in control, and it is a strategy that Navy SEALs use![23] This can be particularly helpful for children who are easily prone to getting frustrated or angry in new situations.

- Remind your child of how a previous situation was handled in a positive way. You can say to the child, "What did you do before? That seemed to work really well." The key is helping children learn to "see themselves" doing what is necessary to remain calm or get through the situation.

- Encourage your child to calm down before attempting to have a discussion about his or her anger/frustration/sadness. Helping your child to be more aware of physical signs or internal dialogues prior to a meltdown, identification of triggers (i.e., baby brother snatched my superhero figurine, a strange dog barked at me, someone cut me in line), and options for calming down are important aspects of later discussions.

- Chunk It: this is an excellent strategy for children to use in many situations. Chunking assignments and just getting through one subject first can reduce the feeling of panic when kids look at a laundry list of homework. Some kids do well when covering rows and rows of math problems so that they only see the first row or one row at a time. When in a stressful social situation, chunking and visualizing getting through small increments at a time can be very helpful and reduces feelings of anxiety.

- Allow for mistakes, especially ones that don't have dire consequences. It's easier to learn from minor mistakes at a young age than costly, serious mistakes at an older age. Reframe the way mistakes are viewed by explaining that making mistakes is inevitable, and that they can be a wonderful opportunity for learning. Many famous inventions were the outcome of mistakes, such as Post-it Notes, Velcro, fireworks, donuts, potato chips, chocolate chip cookies, and ice cream cones, just to name a few.

Physical and Mental Health

There is an old saying that goes, "If you don't have your health, you don't have anything." Of course, the older we get, the more we become aware of the importance of good physical and mental health and wish that we had made better choices when we were younger—eat better, exercise more, meditate, get more sleep, take more vacations, spend more time with family, etc. As parents, you can begin to instill habits for good physical and mental health early on; this will increase the likelihood that your children will practice healthy habits when they are older.

Research shows us that our thoughts and feelings have a strong impact on our physical and emotional health and can actually cause us to heal more or less quickly. Encourage your children to have a positive or optimistic mindset about their mental and physical health. If they are feeling sick, encourage them to visualize themselves feeling healthy and strong. If they are feeling down, encourage them to channel memories of a happier time and to feel those positive emotions.[24]

One way to foster a positive sense of self in your children is to help them find something that they are good at; this will help build their self-esteem. If the child is a good artist, encourage drawing. Perhaps, dance if the child loves music and movement, or a sport if the child has good coordination. Avoid signing children up for an activity that is beyond their developmental skill level, as this could lead to feelings of inadequacy or frustration. Instead, start your children in activities that are suited to their age or ability level that focus on building skills and having fun.

Introduce and encourage your child to listen to music whenever possible; this benefits the brain tremendously and is the brain's equivalent of a full-body workout. It engages practically every area of the brain at once and increases the volume and activity in the bridge between the two hemispheres, which allows messages to travel across the brain faster and through more varied routes.[25] Music can also affect heart rate and blood pressure and can stimulate emotions in the brain and release biochemical materials that change the physiological state. Consider how some kinds of music get you "pumped up" when exercising, while other kinds of music have a soothing effect and might be used to put a baby to sleep.

Another way to boost physical and mental health is to simply go outside and be active in the sun! The heat from the sun affects the endocrine system, which secretes endorphins that are natural chemicals designed to help us relax and feel less stressed.[26] In the summer months, the sun can also be a good source of vitamin D. Recall in chapter 2 that we discussed how salt-filled air near the ocean has a positive impact on our physical well-being; consider placing a salt lamp in an area of your home where people spend a lot of time if you don't live near the ocean.

If you ever question whether your child is in good physical or mental health, before jumping to the conclusion that a child something is wrong and/or requires diagnoses or medication, consider the following:

- "Unplug" children with problematic behaviors from excessive screen time.[27]

- Test your child for food intolerances, allergies, or environmental toxins (consider recent lawn treatments, sensitivities to scents in detergents or skin care products, etc.).

- Consider whether a recent and/or recurring illness (Lyme, strep, earaches, or sinus infections, etc.) could be the underlying cause, and check with a medical doctor to rule this out.

- Some behaviors might be based in a sensory integration problem; an occupational and/or physical therapist can help rule this out.

- Revisit the importance of essential vitamins and minerals to good mental, cognitive, and physical health (discussed in chapter 4).

Communication Skills

Communication involves giving and receiving information and can come in many forms (oral, written on paper, and electronic communication, including social media). Effective communication skills can lead to more successful relationships with family, friends, and/or coworkers. Learning how to communicate with people and for a variety of purposes is an important life lesson. In fact, it's one of the skills that employers value and look for in their new hires. It's never too early to help children learn the art of effective communication:

- Set aside time during the day to be screen free. For example, have screen-free meals and instead enjoy conversation with your family. Time spent in the car is another great opportunity to talk and connect as a family.

- When having a conversation with your children, give them your undivided attention. Getting down on their level, like sitting on the floor or bed, can be helpful. When you do this, you are "telling" them that they matter and are important to you. You are also modeling what active listening looks like, which is 50 percent of good communication.

- Consider asking more open-ended questions, not just "yes" and "no" questions. Some open-ended questions you might ask are:

  o "What did you do at recess today?"

  o "Tell me something that went well today."

  o "I heard about what happened with your friend on Facebook. How do you feel about that?"[28]

- Teach your children how to use an "I message" to communicate feelings. For example, "I feel angry when you call me names. Please stop."

- Make a pact with the parents of your children's friends about the use of cell phones and other important parenting rules and practices. As we discussed in chapter 6, the overuse of cell phones leads to a reduction in good communication skills. Parenting is not easy, especially if you are the one who is trying to be proactive and set reasonable limits and boundaries. If everyone sets similar limits (especially your children's friends' parents), they are easier to enforce.

- Listen more than you talk. Many times, adults feel the need to solve the problem and make it go away, when in fact, your children might just need to talk or "vent" about a problem. The more you listen, the more they will talk, so be patient. Your child might actually solve the problem just by talking about it aloud and with some minimal questioning or commenting from you. Sometimes just a shoulder to lean on, a listening ear, and maybe a hug are all that were needed.

- While parents learn to "pick their battles," so must children. There will always be social situations that just aren't worth the time and energy to engage in or problems worth fixing, and those are the ones that are best ignored, if possible. Sometimes ignoring a situation or annoying behavior or removing oneself from a potentially negative environment or person will be enough. After all, we can't please everyone all the time, or be everyone's friend—and this is important for children to learn over time. However, there will be times when a problem arises within or affects a significant relationship (i.e., a good friend or family member). In those cases, it is important to teach your child that the time and effort are well spent—that avoidance is not the best course of action—because the relationship is worth repairing. Learning effective communication skills is important, but so, too, is knowing when to communicate.

Downtime and Mindfulness

Taking the time to relax and be present in the moment is important and not a waste of time, but in today's overscheduled world it is usually the first thing to go. Allowing daily downtime for yourself and your family is important. It doesn't have to be long, but it is critical to give the body and brain the break they inevitably need. Sometimes the only way busy adults make sure that downtime happens for themselves and their family is by actually scheduling it into the day! How much downtime is enough? There doesn't seem to be a set amount, as everyone is different. However, if you find that you took X number of minutes today or this week, and it didn't seem to be enough to help you feel relaxed and/or recovered from a busy day or week, then you might need a little more downtime.

Allowing daily downtime for yourself and your family is important. It doesn't have to be long, but it is critical to give the body and brain the break they inevitably need. Families have to decide what constitutes downtime for them, but it could include going for a family walk after dinner (no screens), sitting around a fire pit in the backyard and talking, soaking in the bathtub or hot tub, meditating, gardening, or whatever else helps you unwind and relax.

Consider practicing meditation and/or yoga as a way to relax and "clear your brain." "Rest and relax" is a quiet time when your children can be taught to visualize themselves in their favorite calm and peaceful place (a treehouse, a summer vacation spot, their bedroom, etc.). Encourage them to lie in yoga "shavasana" position (flat on their back, arms and legs extended out and eyes closed) and go to that safe place in their imagination. You can play quiet music while they enjoy this downtime. The amount of time that most young children are able to do this is roughly one minute per year of age, so most 6-year olds can enjoy and stay engaged in this type of activity for about six minutes. For children who have great difficulty just "being," gradually build up the amount of time; start with one minute and work your way up. Explain why the activity is important and celebrate when they've done it successfully.

You may also consider devoting one day per week to rest as a family. Perhaps, this could be a family outing to a local park, historical place of interest, a museum, fishing at a local pond, a picnic, watching the weekly football game on Sunday afternoon, or a family activity at home. It could also be hanging by the pool in the summer or having a picnic in the backyard with friends or family. You could even plan the upcoming activity together as a family.

Resilience and Grit

Resilience and grit are two words that often go hand and in hand. The ability to bounce back from life's adversities and the courage to stick with something and see it through to the end are skills that some would say are lacking in young people. However, they are exactly the skills that educators and employers are seeking in their students and employees. That's because psychologists feel that grit is actually a better indicator of future earnings than either IQ or talent. Your child's ability to work hard, persevere, fail, and try again may be the key to long-term success and happiness.[29] To foster grit and resilience in your children, allow them to struggle, feel uncomfortable, and even fail as they learn new lessons and skills. Failure can inspire perseverance and resilience; teach them to deal with disappointment and reframe failure as an opportunity to reflect and learn.

You can also help your children develop a growth mindset rather than a fixed mindset. Individuals with a fixed mindset believe that their intelligence or ability is fixed and cannot change. Studies have shown that teaching people to have a growth mindset encourages a focus on effort rather than intelligence or talent and leads to the belief that it is possible to "grow one's brain." People with a growth mindset believe that intelligence and ability can change and typically become high achievers in school and life.[30] Many schools are now teaching students about the lifelong benefits of having a growth mindset. Phrases that encourage a growth mindset might include: "I'm on the right track," "I'll use a different strategy," "Mistakes help my brain grow," "This may take some time and effort," "Is this really my best work?" or "I am going to take a deep breath and work hard."

To foster a growth mindset throughout your child's life, be sure to praise the process or the effort as much, if not more, than the product. For example, you could say, "I was impressed by the way you kept working until you got the job done," or, "I know how hard you studied for that test. Your effort really paid off!" It is very important that the praise not be connected to a specific outcome, such as an A grade. For example, when students see that a C+ can be praised because it shows improvement over a C−, they will learn to value the work that went into their improvement and will develop a healthy sense of self-worth that is not solely connected to external measures of success like a grade.

Last but not least, encourage your children to engage in physically challenging activities that will require them to persevere through some level of discomfort to achieve a goal. Indoor or outdoor ropes and rock climbing courses are great for this. When children learn that they can struggle and get through discomfort, it is a powerful lesson on perseverance. Keep in mind that it is important to be realistic about your children's physical capabilities and encourage them to participate in activities that are developmentally appropriate.

Problem Solving

Problem solving is a critical life skill and one that is valued by employers. Helping your children become problem solvers encourages independence and autonomy, which are critical to becoming a thriving adult. You don't want your children to always have to call you when they run into a problem. Our job as parents is to help our children become independent and resourceful. Some ways you can do this include:

- Build confidence and competence by offering your child "voice and choice" with choices that are age appropriate and parent approved. For example, you could ask the following questions that presents an opportunity to make a choice:

  o "Would you like to wear your red or blue shirt?"

  o "Do you want to do math or spelling homework first?"

  o "Would you like to play cards or read a story?"

- Don't "rescue" your children too quickly if you see them struggling to solve a problem. Allow time to work through the problem and then offer suggestions if needed.

- Engage in age-appropriate, yet challenging, activities that require persistence and/or a strategy, such as completing a 100- or 500-piece puzzle, checkers, chess, or playing games like Clue, Mastermind, Risk, Operation, and Scrabble.

Cognitive Skills

Cognitive skills allow us to think about and process new information, as well as apply that information to new situations. These skills also include retrieving information from memory, using logic to solve problems, communicating through language, mentally visualizing a concept, and focusing attention when distractions are present.[31] As children mature they improve their ability to think on higher levels, make connections, analyze information, and understand the process of cause and effect. Not only are these skills important for academic success, they can help prevent poor decision-making and giving into peer pressure. When kids can think about the consequence of their actions before they do or don't do something, there can be a more positive outcome. For example, playing video games instead of doing homework can lead to a negative result. While genetics can play a role in cognitive skills, the good news is that they can be taught through experiences and practice. While all children will hit cognitive milestones at different times, if you are concerned about their cognitive development, speak to their pediatrician and/or teacher.[32]

One way to foster the development of cognitive skills is to encourage creative, imaginative play during the early years. You can model imaginative play by encouraging your children to repurpose objects around the house as toys or to use their imagination to create storylines and themes during play. For example, if you use your imagination and creativity, a large cardboard box can turn into a spaceship or time travel machine. Dolls or Lego characters can interact with each other and work together to build a small town, and characters in the town can have their own stories. Furthermore, you could engage in role-play with your young child. For example, you could act out scenarios that might happen in a grocery store, a doctor's office, the post office, or a restaurant, and you could take turns playing different roles (i.e., cashier and customer).

Be sure to avoid introducing skills too early unless your child shows an interest and willingness to learn. This is especially true with writing tasks in the preschool years when many children don't have the fine and gross motor skills to use a writing utensil correctly yet (note, it is much harder to break the habit of the wrong pencil grip then to wait and allow the correct one to develop). Building quantitative skills can be a fun way to lay the foundation for the math curriculum that will eventually come along. For example, take a group of objects (i.e., coins, buttons, shells) and ask your child to sort them by attributes like color, shape, texture, size, purpose, value, etc. After they are sorted one way, you can extend thinking by asking, "How else could you sort them?"

Many parents think it's necessary to accelerate a child's learning by moving to a higher-level reading or math group or even skipping a grade. However, enriching your child's current grade-level curriculum can often be just as beneficial, if not more so, than expanding skills to the next grade level. When parents and educators choose to enrich a child's education rather than accelerate it, deeper levels of understanding and higher-level skills such as application, analysis, and evaluation can be nurtured and developed. Sometimes, "gifted" children (IQ of 130 and above) can potentially handle acceleration, but there may come a point where they are not socially or developmentally ready for the material. A common example of acceleration gone awry is pushing Algebra I down into fifth and sixth grade when the brain may not yet have all the established connections to master abstract concepts. If the foundation for some concepts is weak, this may come back to haunt students when they are in more complex high school–level courses like calculus and physics. With a weak foundation, students may do just average or even poorly in those courses. While it is easy to get caught up in the idea of a student looking very advanced by taking calculus in 10th grade, if the student earned a C this would actually be less impressive to a college admissions counselor than earning an A senior year.

Another great way to enhance learning and cognitive development is through music. Willy Wood, a well-respected educational consultant and coauthor of the book *The Rock 'n' Roll Classroom: Using Music to Manage Mood, Energy, and Learning*, discovered that cognition is enhanced and retention is improved when music is closely connected to learning material. Music that has 60 beats per minute, such as Pachelbel's Canon, is frequently used in classrooms to create a sense of calm and enhance learning, especially during math and writing activities.[33] Movement enhances learning, too. For example, after 15 to 20 minutes of homework, have your child take a movement break or build movement into the actual learning activity. Some kids do better if they can move during studying. You could allow your child to pace or bike on a stationary bike while practicing facts or answering questions, acting out a historical scene when doing history homework, dancing the Macarena to supplement learning multiplication facts, or spelling words while shooting baskets.

For an overall brain boost, consider building Superbrain Yoga into your daily routine.[34] Superbrain Yoga is a specific yoga position. Studies have shown that this specific position results in increased synchronicity between the left and right hemispheres of the brain, boosting numerous cognitive processes. These brain changes have even been captured on EEG in one major study.[35] To achieve optimal results, the position must be practiced daily, but it only takes three minutes! More information can be found in the appendix.

Reading is also critical to cognitive development. If your child struggles with reading, one of the best things you can do is model that reading is enjoyable. If you are seen reading for pleasure, and books are readily available in your home, then your child will learn that reading can be fun. The following are some tips for helping your child overcome reading difficulties:

For Preschool Children

- Begin with small amounts of time. Consider age as a "rule of thumb" for the number of minutes spent reading (i.e., 3-year-old = 3 minutes of time).

- Use short picture books that are engaging and ask questions like, "Can you point to the dog?" or "Where is the bunny?"

- If you child isn't willing or able to sit still on your lap or next to you while you read to him or her, allow the child to stand by you or sit on the floor and listen and look.

- Allow your child to pick the story from a few choices you have preselected. Always include wordless books, easy picture books, alphabet books, rhyming books, and books that stimulate vocabulary.

- When reading, be sure to be animated and use many different voices to engage and maintain your child's focus.

- Start the routine of reading at a very young age. Reading before bedtime provides an enjoyable snuggling time with Mommy or Daddy and helps children calm down and get ready for bed. Of course, there is never a bad time to read with your kids, so anytime that works for your family's schedule is a good time to read!

Elementary and Beyond

- When reading with children, point to the words as you read. As they become readers, they can point while reading to help with tracking and accuracy. There are also strips of cardstock that have a colored acetate strip at the top. This strip goes over the line that the child is reading. It helps with tracking, and for some children the color (especially yellow or blue) can make reading easier on the eyes. See the appendix for more information.

- As children get older, they may prefer nonfiction to fiction books and shorter passages to long chapter books with no pictures. This is when magazines are a great option; reading does not always have to be reserved to books—you can also encourage discovering interesting magazines, news articles, or blogs, and you can establish a routine in which you discuss what they've read about recently. This can be an especially great way to engage with older children.

- Help your children find an interesting or favorite author or series; this can help continue the reading habit at any age.

Meaningful Interactions with Others

Studies indicate that people who have satisfying relationships with family, friends, and the community are happier, healthier, and live longer. Having these meaningful relationships can actually reduce the likelihood of dementia and the harmful and consequential health problems from chronic stress. Caring for others can also cause the release of stress-reducing hormones, so in other words being around people is good for you and your children![36] The following are some ways you can increase or encourage social interactions with and for your children:

- Consider gifts of "time" and "experiences" with your children rather than store-bought gifts. Over the years, gifts are forgotten, but memories will be cherished and shared.

- Help establish playdates or social time for your children. Think of activities like organized sports as being separate from social time. While children are spending time with others during such activities, the time is focused and structured rather than geared toward free interaction.

- Consider donating clothing items (e.g., mittens, coats, or hats) or unused or outgrown toys. When appropriate, children can take their donations to the charity of choice. For example, at holiday time, many churches and schools have food and clothing drives. When children can accompany adults on delivery day, it makes for a meaningful way to actually see how their kindness matters and makes a difference in the lives of others. Even interacting with the sponsors or other volunteers can leave a lasting memory. When children can actually meet the recipients of their kindness that is even better.

- Encourage your children to help trusted neighbors. Perhaps, an elderly neighbor needs help with the yardwork or walking the dog or a lonely neighbor might enjoy some company. Some families open their homes at holiday time and anytime to those who are alone and in need of a friend or a meal. These acts provide experiences early on in life that will nurture kindness and empathy and instill the importance of building meaningful relationships with many different people.

Social Competence

Social competence refers to a person's ability to get along with others. Children are most likely to develop social competence if they feel secure, confident, and if their parents are warm and attentive and also help them understand limits. Social competencies include how to make and be a friend, join a group, compromise, share materials and the "spotlight," and resolve conflicts in a peaceful manner (striving for a resolution that benefits everyone).[37] The following are some ways to enhance social competence:

- Complete jobs around the house; this builds responsibility and helps a child feel like a competent and confident contributor to the family.

- Praise the behavior and character displays you want, and don't just scold the ones you disapprove of.

- As soon as they seem able, encourage your children to speak to teachers, coaches, and other adults on their own behalf. Modeling or role-playing how to do this can be helpful.

- Model responsible use of technology while driving. Hands-free devices offer no safety benefit when driving and do not eliminate cognitive distraction.[38] It is illegal in some states, and if you are doing it, your teenager might think it is okay. There are ways to monitor what your teen driver is doing while driving, but at the very least a family rule about no technology while driving is advisable.[39]

- Consider having a basket for cell phones when kids come over to play or hang out at your house. That way, the kids will be more engaged with each other.

Positive Belief System and Spirituality

We have talked about how a positive belief system, much like a growth mindset, can have positive outcomes on children's physical and mental health, but how about spirituality? Research shows that there are risk factors for children that might cause them to engage in risky behaviors. Likewise, there are protective factors that can help them potentially avoid such things as substance abuse and other harmful actions. Spirituality or religion can have a positive effect on your children.[40] However, beginning in the 1990s and increasing in the 2000s, fewer people affiliated with a religion.[41] Having such a large number of young people disconnected from religion is unprecedented. Regardless of a religious affiliation, the concept of some belief system that believes there is a higher power can help people feel connected, supported, and comforted in times of adversity. The following are some ways that you can harness similar positive effects regardless of whether you consider your family to be spiritual and/or religious:

- Model positive self-talk. If your children see that you believe in yourself and have a positive sense of self, they will adopt that behavior, too. Consider teaching your children to talk to themselves, saying mantras like, "I think I can," "I can do this," "I am brave," or "I've got this."

- Focus on the positive instead of the negative. Denis Waitley, the former head of psychological training for the U.S. Olympic Team, says that many people have a mind full of "ANTs," or abstract negative thoughts, which can have a distracting and even ruinous impact on daily experiences. Waitley teaches athletes to say things like "My muscles are well trained and powerful," rather than "I hope I don't fall." The first statement focuses on the positive, the second thought focuses on the negative.[42]

- Visualize being successful and fulfilling your goals. A brain study on athletes done at UCLA showed that mirror neurons, or neurons that fire during the observation of behavior, lit up while athletes were simply watching videos of themselves.[43] This is an important finding because it indicates that what we see in our minds can translate into our physical reality. If children can "see" or visualize themselves doing something like a dance routine, playing in a soccer match, or making new friends on the playground, the neurons that need to fire while physically doing those things will fire while thinking about them. This starts to help build those neural pathways to make accomplishing the task possible. This can also be done in an academic sense. Children can imagine they are sitting at a desk taking a test and then imagine the answers just coming to them naturally and without stress and worry. Then when they are doing the actual task, they will feel more relaxed and at ease.

- Pair meditation with visualization. Our thoughts house energy that has an effect on us for the positive or negative. Initiate positive meditation and visualization at least once a week. Start with something simple like asking your children what they want for themselves. Young children and even older children who don't have experience doing this may start by listing material things, and this is fine to start. However, try to gradually shift their mindset toward less tangible things. Ask them how they like to feel, and why they like to feel that way. Then tell them to imagine themselves feeling that way. For some children, this may feel overwhelming, so you could instead ask them how they like to see others feel, and why. You can also demonstrate this to them first; you could start by saying, "My hope for you is that you feel happy and loved, because I love X about you." While for some this may feel forced or uncomfortable, over time most children (and adults) come to enjoy this practice and even look forward to doing it!

- If you believe in a higher power, or other spiritual elements, regardless of ties to a specific religion, be sure to share that with your child. Belief in something greater than oneself can provide comfort and strength throughout life's challenges for many people, especially if this is a shared belief in the family.

- Religious institutions often provide volunteer opportunities and support for families. For children who feel less comfortable in large or competitive settings or who are having social challenges in their school setting, they may find a haven in a church or synagogue activity, such as youth group, the children's choir or musical, or faith-based family outings.

Reaching the Pinnacle!

The final block in the pyramid is the pinnacle, the one that all parents hope their child will reach. What a thriving child looks like will vary from family to family. It could include going off to college, obtaining a job in a skilled trade, or becoming an entrepreneur. It could be having a young adult who is happy and healthy, or one who is kind and compassionate and gives to others, or any combination of these milestones and character traits. However, the pinnacle is defined, you want to see your child reach it! Here is one thing we know for sure: life will present challenges and setbacks on the journey to the pinnacle, but it is the way we handle those challenges, the way we frame our thoughts and feelings about them, and how we communicate with ourselves and others about them that will ultimately determine the outcome.

Chapter ten

Interventions and Therapies for When You Need More

"Thought changes structure. I saw people rewire their brains with their thoughts to cure previously incurable obsessions and trauma."

—Norman Doidge, MD

We saved some exciting material for last, but before we share this information, we feel that we have to make you aware of a reality in the world of public education. Many of our readers may be unaware that teachers and school administrators must abide by legal limitations that govern the advice they can provide for pursuing help beyond what the school district offers within the school day. Schools have been subject to lawsuits suggesting that the school cover therapies from which they have said a student could benefit. Therefore, even if school personnel are aware of cutting-edge therapies, they are reluctant to share information about non-school–based therapies or treatment plans because they fear that parents will expect the district to fund these interventions. There needs to be an understanding of therapies and supports that are typically provided by a school district such as basic occupational, physical, and speech and language therapies; services for hearing or vision impairments; and other learning and emotional supports versus those that are outside of the educational umbrella and become the option of the parents to obtain for their child via private insurance coverage or personal funds.

We are going to share therapies and techniques that can be used to help children who are still struggling despite the interventions that have already been tried. Some of these require a recommendation from a doctor, and others can be accessed through a practitioner who has deemed the technique appropriate. Some are paid for by insurance; others are not. If you are not sure if a service is covered, you should start with a call to your insurance provider. Some can be delivered in the school setting, whereas others can be implemented and/or supplemented at home. If you feel like your child is being challenged by something and is not receiving the help that he or she needs or is not making the progress you expected, we hope that this chapter will at least get you started on a path to finding more information and hope!

Note that the information, descriptions, and testimonials that follow are only a brief overview of a variety of interventions and therapies. Please use your own discretion and always consult with your doctor or other qualified professionals to get to the root cause of your child's struggle so that you can pursue the right option(s). Additionally, the highlighted interventions and therapies are by no means an exhaustive list of what is available; we are sure there is even more out there that we have yet to discover!

In an effort to make the information as reader-friendly as possible, we have organized the chapter into general categories broken down by diagnosis, followed by a therapy or therapies that work to address that diagnosis. As you will see when reading the descriptions, some of the interventions or therapies address multiple diagnoses and have been grouped with the diagnosis it may be more commonly known to treat. Please note that the information contained in boxes has been written by a practitioner of the therapy being described, and that sometimes those boxes are followed by text in italics, which have been written by parents of children or individuals who have received the therapy being highlighted. More information and resources can be found in the appendix.

Speech and Language Challenges

Speech and Language Therapy: Many young children have delays or issues in their speech and language development. If your child is slow to develop language and/or has multiple sound errors and is unintelligible to family members and friends, you might want to ask for an evaluation. Many children struggle to enunciate certain sounds, such as: /s/, /z/, /th/, /l/, and /r/. If these are the only sound errors your child is making, the outcome of an evaluation may be to allow more time for those sounds to develop. In any event, the intermediate unit for most public schools provides free evaluations and services for children who have significant delays.

Gross Motor, Fine Motor, and Sensory Integration Challenges

Traditional Physical Therapy/Occupational Therapy: Many young children have delays or issues in developing their fine and gross motor skills. The county intermediate unit for most public schools provides free evaluations and services for children who have significant delays. Many children who have delays or struggles in the area of fine and gross motor skills will not qualify for free services, as they may not be deemed as significantly disruptive. In those instances, you may want to speak to your child's pediatrician and explore whether your private health insurance would provide coverage for sessions, or you could pay for the service out of pocket.

Sensory Integration:[1,2] Sensory integration is a normal, neurological, developmental process that begins before birth and continues throughout life. The most significant "window of opportunity" for development of the sensory system is in the first seven years of life. Sensory processing happens as our neurological system takes in sensory information from the different senses:

Tactile: the sense of touch; input from skin receptors about touch, pressure, temperature, pain, and movement of the hairs on the skin.

Vestibular: the sense of movement; input from the inner ear about equilibrium, gravitational changes, movement experiences, and position in space.

Proprioception: the sense of "position"; input from the muscles and joints about body position, weight, pressure, stretch, movement, and changes in position.

Auditory: input relating to sounds; one's ability to correctly perceive, discriminate, process, and respond to sounds.

Oral: input relating to the mouth; one's ability to correctly perceive, discriminate, process, and respond to input within the mouth.

Olfactory: input relating to smell; one's ability to correctly perceive, discriminate, process, and respond to different odors.

Visual: input relating to sight; one's ability to correctly perceive, discriminate, process, and respond to what one sees.

All of us have preferences when it comes to processing certain sensory stimuli (heavy vs. light touch, smells, food textures, loud noises, bright lights, crowded areas, etc.). Some people need more quiet time or less stimuli to "recharge" and gear up for the next sensory experience, whereas others can keep on going no matter how stimulating their environment is.

When someone's inability to efficiently process sensory experiences significantly impacts developmental skills or everyday functions, then learning, physical and emotional development, and behavior will be impacted. In this case, a sensory processing disorder or sensory integration dysfunction may be present. It is the frequency, intensity, duration, and functional impact of these symptoms that determines dysfunction.

Maude LeRoux, OTR/L, SIPT, RCTC, DIR® Expert Trainer, A Total Approach, fine/gross motor, motor planning, speech, sensory and attention diagnoses

My early work in the United States was with the pediatric population, initially in schools and then in clinical settings. What I observed is that for many children, their intelligence is intact, but somehow their skills did not develop as expected. When school feels overly challenging, children develop the identity of the struggling or anxious learner, or they might try to compensate by developing perfectionist tendencies over things they can do well, or they might put on an air that they don't care. All of this work to cover up insufficiencies drains energy and becomes detrimental to self-esteem. I took a deeper look at what caused children to struggle with fine and gross motor skills, attention, reading, and writing. My research uncovered important information about the brain and body that my staff and I have developed into a model we put into practice with our clients daily. What follows is an oversimplification of a complex process. The autonomic nervous system, composed of the sympathetic and parasympathetic nervous systems, and the sensory system are all tied together. We have 12 cranial nerves in both hemispheres that must gather and make sense of information from our eyes, ears, body, touch, smell, and gravity. A specific timing and homeostasis (ideal balance) must be present within all these various systems for optimal learning to occur. When this homeostasis is not present, children must work much harder than their peers. Children with mismatched and inefficient internal timing or improperly developed sensory systems do not look any different than their peers;

however, they often exhibit difficult behaviors or emotionality because they do not always have the outlet or the language to express their struggles and frustration. Other external signs of these internal challenges might be difficulty cutting with scissors, riding a bike, or doing jumping jacks in unison with peers. They can also have struggles with keeping track of materials, following multistep directions, printing neatly on the lines, or carrying out heavy demand academic tasks such as reading and writing. In my many years of work, I have come to realize that a therapy that only acts on the surface level of a problem may offer temporary relief but often does not offer long-term success. Additionally, the amount and complexity of the challenges children face have increased. Therefore, many strategies that once worked are not enough. This is why we employ brain- and body-based therapies that work with the principle of neuroplasticity, because we can retrain the brain and all the bodily and cognitive processes it controls. It is even possible to identify the earliest points of origin for the dysfunction and to rebuild from the ground up, filling in gaps in development and allowing more complex skills to develop more smoothly. This can be done at any age. We employ the use of reflex integration, deep pressure massage, and a variety of multimodal methods such as Interactive Metronome and Tomatis®. If your child is struggling, I encourage you to "chase the why!"

Brain-Based Therapies for Motor Planning, Sensory Integration, Speech, Attention, and Cognition

Forbrain®: Hearing is a far more complex process than most people realize and involves more than just hearing voices. The brain must be able to make sense of what the ear hears, and this actually involves multiple brain processes. Many bones in the skull and structures inside the ear must work in coordination with the brain for proper hearing and comprehension to occur. If the audio–vocal loop is not working properly for any number of reasons, a lot of verbal information that needs to be taken in is lost, and therefore a real interruption in learning and communication can occur. Forbrain® is a device that has two earbud-like structures that wrap around the outside of the ears but do not sit inside either ear. And, it also has a flexible extension arm that one can place in front of the mouth which both amplifies the wearer's voice and helps filter out extraneous background noise. The buds apply pressure to the bones near the ear, amplifying vibrations and auditory signals. The mouthpiece amplifies the wearer's own voice, allowing the brain to hear the spoken word more clearly. The device also amplifies the voices of those standing in close proximity, allowing the wearer to better comprehend conversations. In a therapeutic setting, the wearer is able to read lessons aloud, which activates other pathways in the brain tied to short- and long-term memory, leading to better retention and recall of learned information. Speech is improved as the wearer is more accurately able to hear his or her own voice. Attention issues also are improved as the filter helps the brain focus on relevant information while blocking out unimportant background noises. The Forbrain® device does not need to be worn all day; it can be worn at home for a small period of time each day. The use of Forbrain® has led to improvement in auditory comprehension, speech annunciation, focus, and long- and short-term memory.[3]

Tomatis®: The Tomatis® Method[4] operates similarly to Forbrain® in terms of how sound activates the brain, but more specifically it acts on the audio-vestibular system. About 80 percent of the stimulation our brain receives comes from the ear! After performing a battery of tests to determine the exact issues, a practitioner can set up a program customized for the child (or teen). The child then undergoes what is called an "intensive," which is a period of 10 to 14 days when a specially designed and programmed headset is worn daily for a 1- to 2-hour block of time. More than one "intensive" may be required to achieve desired results. The sound program offers a huge workout for the brain, via air and bone conduction of the ears and skull, which, in turn, sends a vibration down through the spinal cord, having a strong impact on the vestibular system. The programmed sounds include Mozart (which stimulates the nervous system), Gregorian Chants (which calm the parasympathetic system), and Strauss waltzes (which help the timing of the motor planning system). Some schools in the United States offer Tomatis® as a therapy, but more typically it is done in a practitioner's office. Sometimes a home-based program can be set up. There are even practitioners who will work with you remotely via Skype and rent out the equipment! Tomatis® has helped countless children with attention, learning, emotional, fine and gross motor, and motor planning challenges.

Auditory Processing Challenges

Fast ForWord®: Fast ForWord® is the training program developed by Robert Merzenich and his colleagues, previously mentioned in chapter 2. The program is designed to exercise every brain function involved in language, including decoding sounds and comprehension, which is a more complex reading task that involves integrating many skills at once. Examples of the exercises include teaching children to differentiate between short and long vowels, to differentiate between consonant–vowel combinations that could be confused, and to hear faster and then match sounds to parts of speech. In addition, the exercises teach children to distinguish between consonant sounds such as /b/and /p/ and /d/ and /t/. These are called voiced and unvoiced sounds, meaning they are made with the exact same mouth formations but one is "quiet" and the other is "noisy" and is made by "turning on the motor" or voice box. They can be tricky for young learners. The exercises start off slowly and increase in speed as the child exhibits better grasp of the task. When the child achieves a goal, a reward is flashed on the screen, such as a funny or comical scene. The "reward" is a critical component to the program because when children see something visually pleasing or funny, their brains release neurotransmitters such as dopamine and acetylcholine. Dopamine helps reinforce that something good has happened, and the acetylcholine sharpens the brain's memory of the reward, thus causing the child to want to try again and again, and as we've already shared, the more the child practices skills the more the brain map for that skill develops.[5]

Able Kids Foundation, Fort Collins, CO: At Able Kids, they evaluate and treat clients whose auditory processing difficulties are impacting their lives in school, social situations, relationships, and/or in the work setting. A custom-designed filter device that is clear and small, similar to a hearing aid, is worn in the ear to reduce auditory overload and improve an individual's ability to understand auditory information in difficult listening environments. Unlike the other auditory devices, this can be discreetly worn all day and can be a lifesaver for some children.[6]

> *My child's biggest challenge is his inability to process auditory information. He could barely respond to me in a quiet environment, let alone a busy or chaotic one. I was feeling hopeless, when I heard about a small audiology group called Able Kids in Fort Collins, Colorado. They had a "filter" that could help people with auditory processing disorder. Their auditory testing indicated that the filter would provide benefit for my child, and we have had enormous success with it. They also suggested a FM system in the classroom and time in the day to take 5- to 10-minute auditory breaks. Before the filter, he may not have even known someone was talking to him. With the filter, he now processes, understands, and responds to others. He can attend to his friends on the playground and answer questions in class. His speech therapist and teachers have remarked on how well he does when he is*

wearing his filter. Just the other day, my son was having a very hard time staying on track, responding when spoken to, and was leaving the group (in our relatively quiet home). I asked him if he was wearing his filter. He wasn't. He popped it in and, all of a sudden, he could stay on track and seated for 30 minutes straight. Of all the things we have tried on this journey, Able Kids, their strategies, and their life-changing filter are by far the pieces that have provided the most benefit to my child and my family.

—*Meghan P., Malvern, PA*

If you are unable to access any of the auditory therapies mentioned here for your child, you might consider talking to an official at your child's school about the potential for an FM system in the classroom. Most auditory issues are more complex than simply not hearing well, and an FM system does not work to correct potential brain-based causes of auditory processing issues, but if this is the only help available to a child with auditory processing struggles, it can still have a real impact. The FM system is much like an amplification system, whereby instructors wear a microphone and their voice is projected through a wireless speaker mounted in the room. The students do not have to strain to hear the information, as it is much louder than a normal speaking voice. There is also a model that allows the instructor's voice to be projected directly into an earpiece that is worn by a student.

Visual Processing Challenges

Vision therapy: Being able to see is different than being able to process visual information. A qualified eye doctor can complete an evaluation that goes far beyond looking at the visual eye chart and can let you know if any issue in the visual system could be causing a learning problem for your child.

Dr. Chaya Herzberg, OD, FCOVD, a practitioner of pediatric visual evaluations and therapy

Most children have neither the experience or the language to explain if they have blurred or double vision, so these challenges can often be missed and interfere with learning for years. Children are often prescribed medications for inattention before we check if they can literally focus. I've seen children go through batteries of tests for headaches, including MRIs, before they have a simple eye exam. Many people don't realize that not all eye doctors are the same—it is important to find one who specializes in and understands children's changing needs and development. Eyeglasses are not always required to help a child learn to use and develop their visual skills. Seeing clearly is the first step to understanding, using, and remembering visual information.

Two voluntary muscle systems are involved in our ability to see comfortably. The focusing muscle, within the eye, is responsible for making vision clear at near. The six muscles attached to the outside of each eye are responsible for helping the eyes work together as a team for good depth perception and for moving the eyes in unison for visual tracking. Both systems respond to exercises to increase accuracy and coordination.

Pediatricians and school nurses often check distant vision at 20 feet. But this is not where children learn—they learn from what they can touch, within arm's reach. This is also where they learn to read and write. 20/20 vision, or good vision at distance, does not mean the child has good visual function at near.

Visual feedback is important in the development of fine and gross motor skills. Accurate eye movements are essential for reading, copying and matching. Children need accurate and reliable vision to get the most benefit from physical and occupational therapy. We use pictures and symbols to teach children with speech and language challenges. In other words, good vision is an essential part of learning.

Pediatric optometry is a specialty concentrating on the care of children's vision and the effect of visual dysfunction on learning and development. An evaluation of a child should assess visual acuity or sharpness of sight, refractive error or need for glasses, binocular coordination and depth perception, visual perceptual development, and ocular health.

Until recently, parents were told that children did not require an eye examination until they were ready to enter school. Recent research on infants has shown that many aspects of the visual system mature to adult levels within the first six months of life. We can often prevent impairment and improve function by finding and treating problems early. New techniques enable us to examine the youngest of children. The recommended ages for routine eye care are as follows:

- 6 to 9 months of age for initial examination

- 3 years of age to assure normal development

- 5 years of age to check for school readiness

Your child should achieve certain abilities or skills by a certain age range. Consider consulting a professional for a thorough eye exam if you notice that your infant has difficulty tracking objects, has poor face recognition, and/or eyes that turn in or out; if your preschooler avoids puzzles and manipulatives, has poor eye-hand coordination, exhibits clumsiness, and/or covers or closes an eye; if your elementary school child skips words and consistently needs to reread information, has trouble copying, takes too long to finish work, has poor reading comprehension, complaints of headaches, blurred vision, double vision, and/or exhibits fatigue when reading.

Many of the vision challenges children face respond very well to intervention, and early identification can prevent years of struggling. Possible interventions could include traditional eyeglasses, readers and bifocal eyeglasses, in-office vision therapy, home-based vision activities, and computer-based therapies.

I remember being absolutely terrified in third grade when the teacher asked students to read sections of a book aloud. It was fine when the teacher called upon students in a certain order because I could count the students before me to determine which paragraph I would have to read, then practice my part until it was my turn. Of course, doing this interrupted my ability to pay attention to the rest of the reading or classroom discussion. And, if the teacher skipped around the room and randomly asked people to read, I became incredibly anxious because other students laughed at my attempts to read on the spot. Sometimes, I just got up and went to the bathroom to avoid the humiliation.

For the longest time, I thought it was normal to occasionally see diplopic because I never heard anyone else complain about seeing things blurry; I didn't know it was something to complain about. I, however, did complain about headaches because I would experience them at least four times a week. I also complained about soccer because my vision was so bad on the field I often saw double the players and could not locate the ball. My parents also noticed my aversion to reading and having difficulty locating things around the house. When we met with a pediatric vision specialist, we learned that my symptoms were indicative of a treatable underlying visual perceptual condition.

I started vision therapy, consisting of 30-minute sessions in the vision therapist's office once a week. The therapist programmed activities that focused on my deficiencies in visual memory, laterality and directionality, eye movement skills, focusing, and, of course, eye teaming skills. The muscles that controlled my focus and the muscles that controlled my eye movements were not functioning properly. We used lenses, prisms, red and green filters, and many other pieces of equipment to teach my brain how to properly use my eyes. Other activities focused on teaching my brain how to use information that my eyes brought in. I had a lot of work to do, and many skills that needed development, but we took it one step at a time.

As I developed stronger visual skills, I no longer had to struggle and compensate in other ways in order to keep up with my peers. Once my visual skills were normalized, the barrier to learning was broken, and I felt like I could do anything. My experience was so profound that I decided to become an eye doctor, and I now have the pleasure of helping young people overcome the same challenges I faced.

—Dr. Denise Currier, OD, a practitioner of pediatric visual evaluations and therapy

Reading, Spelling, and Math Challenges

Lindamood-Bell Reading and Math Programs: Lindamood Bell is a company that was founded in the 1970s by Pat Lindamood and Nanci Bell. Their philosophy has always been that all individuals, including those with dyslexia, ADHD, and autism, can learn. Lindamood Bell programs include the following:[7]

- **Talkies®:** Develops sensory-cognitive processing for the imagery-language connection for students of all ages and ability levels.

- **Lindamood Phoneme Sequencing®:** Develops phonemic awareness, or the ability to identify the number and sequence of sounds within words; this supports accurate and confident decoding and spelling.

- **Visualizing and Verbalizing (VV) for Language Comprehension and Thinking®**: Develops oral and written language expression, comprehension, concept imagery (the ability to create an imaged gestalt/whole from oral and written language), and critical/analytical thinking.

- **On Cloud Nine Math®**: Develops numeral and concept imagery to improve mathematical concepts and computation.

- **Seeing Stars®**: Develops symbol imagery or the ability to visualize sounds and letters within words, in order to improve visual memory, word attack, word recognition, spelling, and contextual reading (both accuracy and fluency).

Lindamood Bell has partnered with many universities to study the positive effects of their programs on brain development. These studies have shown significant positive brain changes, including increased gray matter volume in the areas of the brain that have been shown to play a part in learning and visual imagery, and improved reading skills and brain changes were maintained after the instruction ended.[8]

The latest study was completed during the summer of 2017 under the leadership of Jason D. Yeatman, an assistant professor of speech and hearing sciences at the University of vWashington. Julie Gunter, parent of a child with dyslexia, partnered with Yeatman and Lindamood Bell to access Seeing Stars instruction for her daughter. Incredibly, after just eight weeks of therapy, Gunter reported that her daughter's reading fluency jumped two grade levels due to the intensity and quality of instruction, her youth, persistence, and desire to learn. Gunter states, "While our daughter was extremely fortunate to receive this life-changing intervention, I'm keenly aware that other children who struggle with learning to read due to dyslexia (whether diagnosed or not) may never receive the type of instruction that could make a transformative difference in their lives."[9] Yeatman states, "One thing I can say definitively is that the intensive reading intervention program changes the underlying structure of the brain. That's something that we're clearly seeing."[10]

Lindsay LaRiviere, MEd, Lindamood Bell Center Executive Director, Bryn Mawr, PA

At Lindamood-Bell, we believe all students can learn to their potential. We believe sensory cognitive functions support language and literacy development, and we know, through experience and research, that our unique approach to instruction allows for students to make significant progress in reading and comprehension. However, a few big things have changed since the first program was originally created. Prestigious universities have utilized our programs to show changes in the brain for students diagnosed with dyslexia and autism. We are able to offer the same research validated instruction to students in any corner of the globe with our virtual model, and we now have our own accredited K-12 school, Lindamood Bell Academy. All students who walk through our doors have their own story, their own measure of success. For some it's foundational reading skills, and for others comprehension at a college level. For some students, the academic goal is in between. Our goal is to create the magic that not only lets them read and comprehend to their potential but also to give them the confidence to strut out of our learning center. As our founder, Nanci Bell, would say, "Lucky us!"

When my son and daughter were headed into third and second grade, both were reading very far below grade level and were frustrated, embarrassed, and hated school. After learning about Lindamood Bell through one of their teachers, I took a look at their website, and it quite literally brought tears to my eyes. Everything about the Lindamood Bell approach, the research behind what they do, and the stories from other parents felt like someone finally understood what we were going through. That feeling carried through our initial evaluations, which gave us a specific plan to help them. In our case, the plan was based on the Seeing Stars program. At the Learning Center, the children flourished. It was hard work for them for four hours a day, five days a week, but they left that center happy every day. The Lindamood Bell instructors understand how beat down these children feel, and they are well trained to provide not only the right instruction but the right attitude and energy to help the children walk away with real confidence in their own abilities. I am truly grateful to have found Lindamood Bell.

—*Michelle R., Kennett Square, PA*

Attention Deficit Disorder/Attention Deficit Hyperactivity Disorder

Neurofeedback

Neurofeedback teaches the brain to change itself and has been shown to improve attention, mood, behavior, and cognition. An initial full brain EEG, or brain map, is taken to study the brainwaves and patterns of that person's unique brain. Presuming areas of weakness are found (meaning non optimal brainwave patterns in various parts of the brain), those areas of the brain can be trained via neurofeedback to work more efficiently. A new full-brain EEG can be taken following treatment to show the progress the treatment has made. Neurofeedback has been used to treat ADHD, ADD, anxiety, phobias, sleep disorders, addictions, post-concussion syndrome, seizures, and more.[11]

Holly Grimm, LCSW, and Todd Grimm, LPC, board certified practitioners in neurofeedback

The brain can be divided into two parts: a part that is under our direct control and a part that functions automatically outside of our control. Most people seek help in therapy due to thoughts and feelings that belong to this second category. They "know" how they should think or feel, but they can't seem to change those thoughts or feelings. For example, a person may "know" that an airplane is a relatively safe mode of transportation, but when they try to get on the airplane, automatic negative thoughts in their mind begin, and they can become very frightened. Traditional therapy seeks to use the part of the brain that is under our direct control to attempt to influence the part that functions automatically. While it can be very effective, used alone it can take long periods of time to affect change, as this change occurs by indirect means. In the case of biologically related conditions such as ADHD, permanent change must often be maintained through a structured pattern of living, which can include employing continued thought restructuring and organizational techniques. Years ago, when we started learning about neurofeedback, we realized that it could bypass the part of the brain under our direct control and work directly on the automatic part of our brain, similar to psychotropic medications. We've noticed that the change can be much faster than with therapy alone, and for biologically based conditions it often provides a solution that does not require long-term work or maintenance on the part of the client. However, unlike medications, neurofeedback only has mild initial side effects for some, which are similar to those one experiences when practicing meditation, and creates lasting improvements, even after treatment has stopped. In fact, in a 1995 study about 80 percent of people who had neurofeedback substantially improved symptoms of ADD/ADHD, and these gains were maintained 10 years later. Of course, it takes time to get to that level of improvement; neurofeedback requires a twice weekly time commitment for approximately 30 to 60 sessions for most people to achieve their desired results, with some occasionally needing more sessions depending upon a number of factors. It is also important for people engaging in neurofeedback to realize that they can help it to work faster by creating healthy lifestyle habits. In our years of doing neurofeedback, even without significant work to modify thoughts or behaviors, we've seen it help people to significantly decrease anxiety, phobias, and depression, and to help people (even post-concussion) to focus better, improve their memory, get better sleep, and increase skills such as reading, handwriting, and drawing. From these changes, we've seen people's self-esteem increase, levels of happiness and success rise, and families heal. Neurofeedback has been designated a "Level 1 Research—Best Support Intervention" by the American Academy of Pediatrics and is also one of the most effective, efficient, and side-effect–free tools we have used to help people rise to their potentials.

When I attended my son's kindergarten conference, I left feeling discouraged and overwhelmed. The teachers described his difficulty paying attention, staying on task, and following directions. I contacted the guidance counselor, and she began an assessment and classroom observations. I took all of that data to the pediatrician. He confirmed what everyone suspected; my son had ADD. The doctor spoke to us about the possibility of medication, but I wasn't ready to take that step. I remembered that a friend had posted something on Facebook about a local psychologist who was using neurofeedback to address ADD. I contacted the psychologist, and my son was evaluated and given an EEG. The psychologist reviewed the results and told us she believed neurofeedback could help our son. He began therapy the next week. Within three sessions, I noticed a significant improvement in his handwriting. We continued the sessions for a while, and by the time I attended his first-grade conference, the transformation was unbelievable. His first-grade teacher stated that if she hadn't been told he had ADD, she may not have picked up on it. He is now in third grade and has excellent grades and functions very well in the classroom.

—Emily M., parent of a third grader

Interactive Metronome (IM)

The brain has an internal "clock" that keeps time for various systems. This time is kept in seconds, milliseconds, microseconds, etc., depending on the function. The brain has a kind of timing called temporal processing that involves neurons firing in precise timing; it is responsible for detecting sound and regulating attention and many other cognitive functions. A growing amount of research suggests that there is a deficit in this system for children who have ADD, ADHD, dyslexia, and autism, etc. Interactive Metronome (IM) aims to train the brain to get that internal clock and timing system working correctly through a series of computer-simulated activities that offer the brain and body immediate feedback. By participating in this training over a period of time, the body gets back in sync with its own internal clock, thus either greatly reducing or even eliminating many of the struggles that come with the above-listed diagnoses.[12]

Our son was diagnosed with attention deficit disorder. He seemed a bit "lazy" when it came to his work and disliked reading immensely. When we met with our college consultant at the end of his junior year, she was surprised by his SAT scores given her interaction with him. She suggested that we get him retested academically since the last time had been in third grade. We did and discovered his aptitude was quite high (verbal IQ of 134) but his processing speed was not, creating a much bigger gap between the two since the last evaluation. Since time was so critical at this stage, we took her advice to use the Interactive Metronome therapy, which included 16 one-hour sessions over the summer.

His GPA rose from a cumulative 3.2 through junior year to a 3.6 for the first half of senior year. In addition, his SAT scores rose nearly 300 points. However, the biggest change I noticed was that my son felt smarter, understood himself and how he uniquely learns better, and became highly motivated to achieve —he was admitted to a great college, has acclimated well, and even got an A- in calculus!

Because of my son's results, we engaged IM therapy for our daughter when she began to struggle academically as a high school freshman. Her difficulty was more in the area of math and language. IM has improved her ability to retrieve and manipulate data, which has been a struggle for her. The biggest advantage of IM for me as a parent is the permanent change that occurs in a child's brain. It is not a therapy that must be continued to be effective. The positive results are lasting. Although the therapy is not inexpensive, it is much less costly than a drug-dependent solution without any negative side effects.

—Grateful parent

We have highlighted a number of interventions and techniques that work on the brain and body to help children with learning struggles learn better. If these are inaccessible to you due to your location or finances, consider talking to your school administration about the following revolutionary program that has been designed for schools to help all children have a more enriching and effective school experience. It has been implemented in over 3,400 schools worldwide.

Action Based Learning

Dr. Jean Blaydes Moize, founder and practitioner of Action Based Learning (ABL) and professional training director and innovations writer for Kidsfit

Action Based Learning is based on brain research that supports the link of movement with improved learning. The latest research in neuroplasticity and epigenetics says that the brain can and does change, and we can influence positive change to foster better brains for our children.

Activities in the Action Based Learning ABL Labs are designed to intentionally fill in developmental gaps to prepare the young brain for learning. Brain science and child development tell us that certain foundations are needed for the brain and body to work in concert for improved learning. Developmental gaps can delay learning, but neuroplasticity allows us to change the brain by using specific movements like crossing the midline or improving gross motor skills. The Action Based Learning Lab is based on these basic Foundations and provides activities to support all:

Cross the Midline: Cross Lateralization
Body in Space: Vestibular Balance Spatial Awareness
Balance: Spatial Orientation
Visual Development: Encoding Symbols
Rhythm: Beat Awareness Beat Competency
Tactile Learning: Sensory Motor and Fine Motor Skills
Motor Skills: Locomotor and Nonlocomotor
Coordination: Manipulative Skills
Physical Fitness: Strength and Flexibility
Cardiovascular Health
Problem Solving: Embodied Cognition
Self-Management: Mindfulness and Self Awareness

Action Based Learning strategies and activities blend academics with movement to increase learning and are designed with developmental ages in mind. There are labs for PreK–2nd grade, 3rd–5th grades, and 6th–12th grades.

Emotional Challenges

Individuals who may have already had a number of negative life experiences that have been reinforced in their mind, or who have not gotten good results from traditional talk therapy, might consider seeing a psychologist who practices techniques such as Neuro Emotional Technique (NET), Eye Movement Desensitization and Reprocessing (EMDR), or Emotional Freedom Technique (EFT). These techniques are aimed at restoring balance to the mind–body connection, and in a sense, "erasing" the body's automatic memory that can kick in when the child (or adult) encounters certain triggers or triggering situations that are likely brought on due to some type of past trauma.

Neuro Emotional Technique (NET)

The objective of NET is to help clients become less physically reactive to distressing stimuli and to become more capable of choosing alternative responses. A recent study done at Thomas Jefferson University found that NET can reduce the symptoms of traumatic stress in cancer survivors. Functional MRI studies conducted before and after NET showed significant and substantial changes in the brain and in a short period of time. Every single patient in the study reported feeling better after NET, and for some even three to five sessions resulted in feelings of significant improvement. One of the researchers used the saying that "a picture is worth a thousand words," and while clinical evidence is important, seeing the physiological changes in the brain speaks volumes.[13]

Dr. Christine Hannafin, licensed psychologist and practitioner of NET

NET draws on a combination of principles from psychology, neuroscience, and acupuncture theory. Emotions are signals, indicating how things are going for us in life. Different chemistry is present as various emotions are experienced. The emotions are to serve us, and when various needs are met, nature intends for that chemistry to subside. However, if a person has experienced an emotional or physical trauma, the body may not have discharged this chemistry, and it can be retriggered, by similar stimuli, in an unconscious, conditioned process. The presence of this chemistry can cause a blockage of the electrical flow of the body, causing physical pain, illness, or emotional distress. Muscle testing is utilized to determine the origins of the blockage, clear it and allow the energy to flow. This unhooks conditioned responses, enabling a client to feel and/or behave in a more effective manner.

Eye Movement Desensitization and Reprocessing (EMDR)

EMDR is a form of psychotherapy pioneered by Dr. Francine Shapiro in the late 1980s to treat posttraumatic stress disorder, as well as traumatic experiences in general. More than 50,000 psychologists in the United States are now using this technique. EMDR therapy is recommended as an effective treatment for posttraumatic stress disorder in the practice guidelines of a wide range of organizations, including the American Psychiatric Association (2004), the Department of Veterans Affairs and Department of Defense (2010), the International Society of Traumatic Stress Studies (2009), and other organizations worldwide. The goal of EMDR is to lessen the power that traumatic memories have over our brain. The practitioner will work through a traumatic memory with patients by asking them to visualize or recall difficult memories while asking them to simultaneously move their eyes in a rhythmic, but rapid, side-to-side fashion, typically while following an instrument that is being moved back and forth in front of the patient's eyes. The swift eye movements are believed to "loosen knots" in one's memory and allow negative thoughts and memories to be reprocessed into new, nontraumatic thoughts.[14]

Emotional Freedom Technique (EFT)

Suzanne Rossini, certified EFT practitioner

EFT, or "tapping" as it is commonly known, is a somatic/cognitive modality also known as a form of emotional acupressure. Its foundation is based on the knowledge that energy flows through the body in patterns. In ancient Chinese medicine, these energy channels are called meridians. In theory, negative emotions disrupt these patterns, resulting in all kinds of undesirable responses, both physical and emotional. The amygdala is the stress alarm of the body; it triggers the fight-flight-freeze response when it perceives we are in danger or that a threat is present and triggers the release of stress hormones, cortisol and adrenaline. In terms of trauma, the amygdala is on overdrive, due to the limbic system constantly perceiving anything that resembles the original trauma as an immediate threat. "Tapping" on acupressure points while "talking" about a specific problem sends a calming signal to the amygdala, via the body's energy meridian system, resulting in a sense of overall calm and clarity. The" talking" (cognitive) part of EFT targets the problem and the "tapping" (somatic) part changes the behavior or perception. Tapping also resets the hippocampus, the memory part of the brain, which compares past threats with present signals and tells the amygdala whether a threat is actually present. It is important to understand that there are two forms of EFT: clinical and self-care. Clinical EFT requires a practitioner to guide the client through the core issues that have been obstacles to healing. These issues can range from limited beliefs to unresolved traumas that have resulted in unhealthy and self-defeating behaviors. Often clients are unable to make these connections on their own. Remember, the events that created your belief system have specific details that are uniquely yours. Those details are used in individual sessions to get to the heart of the matter.

Sadly, on December 14, 2012, one of the worst school shootings took place at Sandy Hook Elementary School in Newtown, Connecticut. The Newtown Trauma Relief Project (NTRP) developed through the efforts of Dr. Lori Leyden, PhD, MBA, and internationally known stress and trauma healing expert, Nick Ortner, Newtown resident and CEO of The Tapping Solution, and Scarlett Lewis, mother of 6-year-old Jesse, who lost her life that day. The mission statement of NTRP was to empower the community to heal from the trauma and suffering from the Sandy Hook tragedy using leading-edge modalities for trauma and PTSD, both long and short term. Scarlett Lewis, Founder of the Jesse Lewis Choose Love Movement, is quoted as saying,

> Although we can't always choose what happens to us, we can always choose how to respond. Children can learn to choose a loving thought over an angry one. When a child realizes that they have the power to positively impact themselves as well as those around them, it is empowering and perpetuates their positive actions and interactions.[15]

Tapping has proven to be an effective therapy to combat the effects of such a traumatic event. Eric Leskowitz, MD, of the Department of Psychiatry at Harvard Medical School states,

> Based on my clinical experience and reading of the research literature, EFT/Tapping is the treatment of

choice for rapid intervention in traumatic situations like Newtown, that trigger overwhelming emotions in individuals and groups. Its use can prevent future development of full-blown PTSD by empowering people to develop control over their own nervous system.[16]

Educators and parents are finding that tapping is a lifelong skill that can be used by anyone who is experiencing anxiety or suffering from the effects of past trauma.

EFT, or Tapping, is an extraordinary way to relax, focus, release anxiety, and integrate positive thoughts into one's day. It has created a significant transformation with my teaching and student learning. The dynamics of the room change when students begin to tap. They become quiet and focused through the process, releasing first negative thoughts and then replacing them with positive, self-enriching ones. A wonderfully calming and centering technique, tapping allows us to move through the lesson with minimal disruption. Tapping has also created a sense of safety and community in our classroom. It is a form of stress relief that is a straightforward and a viable method to improve student behavior, academics, and classroom management. It has also given students a sense of personal responsibility and autonomy, in that they have more control over their personal actions and reactions.

Tapping helps my students when they are in class, but also when they leave the classroom. Many take tapping with them, and if feeling overwhelmed, anxious, or sad, they have a tool to help calm themselves. One high school student told me, 'When I see that there is homework on the board, I know I will have to stay up late to finish it. I start to tap, even though I don't notice I am. Then I feel that anxious feeling go away.' Another student who sets high expectations for herself and is involved in many extracurricular activities shared,

"When I tap, I take my mind off of the pressure life holds on me. I can finally breathe. I am so thankful to have learned this method in middle school. Thanks to a wonderful teacher, I am able to become a happier and healthier person. Tapping has positively changed my life for the better. I will continue to tap and share it with my friends and family for years to come."

Many of my students choose to teach their parents and siblings, which reinforces community within their homes. I am so grateful to have been introduced to this method, not only for the integrity of my classroom, but for my students, their families, and me. Through 34 years of teaching special and general education, I have found tapping to be one of the most meaningful teaching tools I have ever used.

—Moira, MEd, sixth-grade teacher

Other Physical and Mental Health Challenges

The following approaches are intended to foster overall wellness of brain, body, and in some cases, even spirit. These would all be accessed outside of a school setting, but for some can have a powerful impact on all arenas of one's life.

Integrative Medicine

This type of medicine offers a comprehensive look at health and wellness. Integrative medical doctors are interested in understanding the root cause of the symptoms their patients are experiencing. These doctors use a broad array of diagnostic testing to identify the cause of symptoms, considering factors such as nutrition, immune deficiencies, and the environment, which can contribute to neurochemical imbalances and general inflammation of the body and brain.[17, 18] For doctors to hold integrative medical credentials, they must engage in significant training beyond their initial medical degrees. Integrative medical doctors incorporate the best of traditional medicine with well-researched alternative practices and techniques.

Epigenetics

This is an evolving specialty area that recognizes that the genes we are born with cannot change, but they can change their expression, being turned on and off not by the genes themselves, but in response to external stimuli. Stimuli could be the assault of an illness (bacteria, virus, fungi, or parasites) or even a traumatic experience that is psychological in nature. Many specific genes have been identified and their mechanisms understood. Researchers, scientists, and doctors have discovered and continue to discover ways to heal the body using their understanding of epigenetics.[19]

As an example, researchers and doctors working in the field of epigenetics have made important discoveries about a pathway called the methylation pathway. This is a biochemical pathway that is involved in most bodily functions, managing or contributing to detoxification, immune function, energy production, mood balance, and the control of inflammation. Researchers have learned a great deal about specific genes in this pathway from which parents of children with chronic health or learning, behavioral, or emotional problems could benefit.

For example, genes have been identified that impact how much vitamin D makes it into our cells. Vitamin D is critical to a strong immune system, so when these gene mutations are triggered, one is more prone to immune-related health issues. Genes also control the production and utilization of serotonin. If these genes are not expressed properly, depression and attention and sleep disturbance could result. Genes also regulate dopamine production, and when not expressed properly, ADD/ADHD or other diagnoses, such as Parkinson's, can be the outcome. Genes have been identified that control epinephrine and norepinephrine production. When these genes are not expressed properly, bipolar and conduct disorders can be a result. Doctors who understand this pathway can run tests to look at neurotransmitter function. Many conditions, such as ADD, autism, and a broad variety of autoimmune illnesses, have been treated by using specific supplements that support the correct and efficient function of the methylation pathway.[20]

> Our integrative medical doctor taught us many things to help us understand our daughter's immune system. She ran a number of tests that provided helpful information and created an alternative treatment plan that consisted of a team of well-trained practitioners. We learned we had some problematic genes that had been turned on. For some reason, this information didn't scare us but empowered us and provided an explanation for what had happened, and most importantly, it offered us a plan for healing. The nutrigenomic protocol we followed was based on our daughter's specific weaknesses within that pathway. There are known supplements, which help make up for the body's inability to function properly. We were encouraged to introduce one supplement at a time to allow her body to adjust. Some of the supplements do cause the body to release deeply held toxins, so the adage, "it can get worse before it gets better," sometimes applied. When the body begins to release toxins and heal, there can be rashes, or sleep disturbance, and sometimes even fevers, but our doctor helped us understand that this was a normal healing reaction. It did take three years of careful supplementation for our daughter to heal,

but when you look at how ill she was, this was a child facing a feeding tube and who could not tolerate any real food. This was a child who had virtually no immune system to protect her, and we almost had to live in a bubble and isolation to keep her safe. Now this child is thriving and healthy. Was the journey sometimes hard? Absolutely. But with the right team and attitude, you can do it. When we first started this journey over a decade ago, there were few doctors in the country who understood methylation, nutrigenomics, and the overall genetic research. Now, there are actually many integrative or functional medical doctors who do. Our daughter's situation was extreme; however, as a family we have all become stronger from what we learned, and we have seen children with lesser issues recover much more quickly than our daughter did.

—Monica and Rob

Nutritional Response Testing (NRT)

Dr. Nathalie Matte, DC, and NRT practitioner

Nutritional Response Testing (NRT) is a very effective and non-invasive system that uses acupressure points and muscle reflexes to identify areas of disease in the body. The acupressure points are selected from ancient Chinese systems of acupuncture. Once issues have been identified, a tailored, specific nutritional program with appropriate supplements is drawn up for the patient. This will provide them with the exact nutrients they need to improve their health. The system is designed to prioritize health issues through its own innate intelligence. The body has a natural inborn intelligence or order of survival. It's the body's ability to self-regulate, self-heal, and self-adapt if it has no interference.

A chiropractic patient of mine had been coming in for chiropractic adjusting for quite some time, and every visit I noticed redness on the skin under her eyebrows. We did NRT testing and discovered that she had high levels of formaldehyde in her body due to frequent contact with the chemical each day at work. We had her do a detoxification supplement program and the rash quickly disappeared. We must remember that the skin is our largest organ in the body, and sometimes it tells us when something is not right on the inside. I have had several rash cases over the years, and they normally clear up very easily as we address the cause. Identifying the cause is the important part.

Chiropractic Care

Many people are under the impression that chiropractic care is only for adults and for people who are trying to recover from an injury, but, in fact, chiropractors regularly work with children and often adjust newborn babies!

Dr. Janet McGaurn, DC, chiropractor

The central nervous system (CNS) controls and coordinates every organ, system, and tissue of the body. Every cell of the body has a direct link to the CNS. The CNS is composed of the brain and the spinal cord. The spinal cord has nerve roots that send and receive nerve signals to every cell of the body. This system is the most vital system of the body, and because of this nature designed that it be completely protected by bone, with the bones being separated into segments so that we can move and twist and bend. When the vertebra line up correctly, it allows the hole created by the perfectly aligned vertebra to be wide enough for the nerve roots that exit the spine to send and receive signals to and from the body without any interference. The one flaw in the protection provided by the need to bend, twist, and move is the vertebral subluxation. A vertebral subluxation occurs when the body is overwhelmed by stress in any form (spiritual, mental, emotional, chemical, or physical) and a vertebra becomes misaligned with the vertebra above and below it. This causes pressure to be exerted on the nerve root. Pressure on the nerve root interferes with the communication between the brain and the organs, systems, and tissues that are supplied with this vital communication at the level of the subluxation. Chiropractors gently and specifically adjust the vertebra back into place to relieve the pressure on the nerve roots, and this allows the body to function at its highest potential. Chiropractic is much more about overall health and well-being and the proper functioning of the entire body and much less about aches and pains. With the advent of children and teens using multiple devices for school, homework, and other activities, the amount of time that the cervical spine (neck) is placed in flexion (looking down at these devices) has caused a straightening or complete reversal of the cervical curve that is usually seen after trauma such as automobile accidents, serious falls, and sports injuries to name a few. Chiropractic adjustments help to correct this along with teaching children and teens how to change their posture and hold or change where these devices are placed to minimize the strain on the cervical spine.

Acupuncture

Acupuncture is a form of traditional Chinese medicine that has been practiced for centuries. It is based on the theory that there are energy channels that run throughout the body, and recall from chapter 2 that modern science has confirmed that the body does create electrical energy that can be measured. Practitioners refer to this energy as "chi" (pronounced "chee"). Acupuncturists believe that illness is experienced when there are blockages in energy channels, so they carefully insert very thin needles into specific pathways to unblock the energy flow. Acupuncture has been used to treat a broad variety of health ailments such as morning sickness, concussions, vertigo, pain relief, allergies, migraine headaches, and dental pain and for improving sleep.[21]

Note that EFT, discussed earlier in this chapter, is based on the same principles of blocked energy in the body's meridians. Other techniques that are born of this concept, but do not use needles like acupuncture does, are acupressure and reflexology. These techniques can be used on children and even babies.[22]

Homeopathy

This is yet another treatment methodology that operates on our body's energetic system.

Peter Prociuk, MD, licensed doctor, and practitioner of classical homeopathy

In the late 1700s, Dr. Samuel Hahnemann, the founder of homeopathy, was fervently looking for a method of healing that worked with the natural healing powers inherent in every living creature. His daughter had recently died as a result of the conventional treatments of the day, and he was determined to discover a better way of treating the sick. He founded a system of energy-based medicine based on a law of nature more than 100 years before the discoveries of Albert Einstein. While researching the action of medicines, he consumed a larger than usual amount of *Cinchona officinales* tincture, a rainforest tree used at the time for treating malaria, and it produced the symptoms of that disease—high relapsing fevers, profound weakness, and drenching sweats. This quandary, how an effective medicinal substance produced the likeness of an illness in a healthy man, which it cured in one afflicted with the disease, provoked much more research. Through many experiments and meticulous observation, he discovered a fundamental law of nature, which governed the response of living organisms to medicinal substances. To implement this law into a comprehensive medical science, Hahnemann had to discover how herbal, mineral, and animal derived medicines acted. He conducted many meticulous experiments to discover the symptoms so produced, and this became the basis for the current Homeopathic Materia Medica.

Homeopathy is based on using medicines whose actions are similar to the illness. This is in direct contrast to conventional medicine where medicines act opposite to the action of the illness. Hahnemann was the first physician to clearly understand that only a similar medicine can arouse a curative response, whereas using opposite medicines only results in the suppression of symptoms. We now have well over 1,000 remedies whose action is known well enough to use effectively. Hahnemann's goal was to discover the minimum dose required to arouse the healing instinct. The basis for this was that all functions of a living organism in health or illness are determined by the vital force (chi in Chinese Medicine) within it. The physical changes in a sick patient result from a disturbed vital force and to correct it required medicines that were vital, or energetic, in nature.

A simple example is a light bulb in which the current is faulty. No matter how much the bulb is adjusted it will not function correctly until the current is corrected. Hahnemann's concept of dose, or potency as it's called in homeopathy, was the stimulus needed to arouse patients to heal their own "current." He discovered how to extract the energetic nature of a medicine and reliably administer it. Today homeopathic remedies are legally categorized as drugs, must be made in licensed pharmacies by licensed pharmacists, and are regulated by the FDA. Homeopathy can be used effectively in a wide range of conditions in every age group.

When I was about 12 years old, I had a chronic sinus infection for about two years. I struggled throughout the day with the constant pressure in my head. I visited multiple doctors, tried antibiotics, daily sinus rinses, but nothing worked. I finally underwent a sinus and adenoid surgery. I thought that had cured me, yet after just three days, my sinuses were again congested, and I felt hopeless. At that point, my mom, who was a lifelong nurse, remembered a note one of the recovery room nurses had slipped to her after my surgery that said, "call him when your son's sinus infection comes back" and had the name of a local homeopathic doctor.

My mom made an appointment. Instead of scoping me up the nose or down the throat, the long and uncomfortable procedure I was used to receiving, this new doctor simply asked me questions about my favorite foods, my hobbies, and my personality traits. After about a half hour of interrogation he said, "I know just the remedy to cure you." He explained that instead of trying to cure the sinus infection directly, the remedy would help build up my immune system to fight off the infection through its own natural process. I left the appointment feeling skeptical, but after about a week or so, my sinus infection began to subside, and eventually was completely gone. Additionally, other issues I had been struggling with like anxiety and occasional bed wetting had completely disappeared. I couldn't believe that all I needed was one simple remedy to help me live a normal, healthy life.

—Matthew, 18 years old, freshman at Dartmouth University

Conclusion

"Never doubt that a small group of thoughtful, committed citizens can change the world. Indeed, it is the only thing that ever has."

—Margaret Mead

Throughout our book, we have touched on many reasons why today's world is different, how things introduced into our environment have had an impact on children and the way they function, and why the education system in America is challenged. Despite some of this disheartening information, we believe that all children have an innate desire to learn and the potential to thrive in the classroom and beyond. The culprits we've highlighted can rob children of natural learning opportunities, as well as alter the way their brains and bodies function, but this is where we can take back some of the control by implementing limitations and introducing helpful strategies. With purposeful parenting and by keeping the culprits in check, the building blocks in the pyramid model we introduced in chapter 9 will naturally fall into place, leaving opportunities for critical lifelong skills to develop.

There was a poem written many years ago by Joseph Malens, entitled "An Ambulance Down in the Valley." It talks about a town that had once engaged in a very bitter debate about whether the best way to deal with the problem of people falling off a local cliff high above the city was to raise funds to build a fence at the top of the cliff or to continue to raise funds to park an ambulance down in the valley, which was very efficiently hauling people off to the hospital. A lot of the townspeople said, "Look, we've always had an ambulance there and it's worked very well. Why should we raise more funds to build a fence?" But finally, common sense prevailed. Someone stood up and said, "An ounce of prevention is worth a pound of cure."[1]

Currently, the prevailing models for education and health in our country are ones focused on treatment rather than prevention. We would like to see a shift toward wellness and prevention, but we can't just talk about it—we have to take action. So how can we take action? On a small scale, we can start by taking a look within our own homes and by asking ourselves if and how we can make improvements in the areas of daily life presented in this book—improvements in our family's diet or physical environment, in the way we allocate time to activities like play, or to technology like phones and computers. We can reflect on the way we interact with our children and consider the impact that our parenting style has on our children's development. Then if we can identify areas that need improvement, we can implement strategies like those presented in this book.

On a larger scale, we need to get involved in our communities and grassroots efforts aimed at improving our knowledge, our culture, and the environment regarding children and their mental and physical health. For example, Dr. Kathy Hirsh-Pasek founded a movement called, "The Ultimate Block Party," which are well-organized, scientifically supported, locally held events aimed at getting parents and kids out to play.[2] Or consider following groups like Documenting Hope that offer parents many free resources and a place to start in learning about various physical and mental health diagnoses, as well as underlying causes and treatments.[3]

We can also use our voting power to support local, state and national representatives who prioritize children's issues. Our voices can make a difference. Some large food corporations are starting to change the way they make foods by pulling out or reducing controversial ingredients, dyes, and additives. Concerned consumers forced this to happen by buying less of the bad stuff and more of the good. Also, demand for healthier and more affordable food options has led to the creation of companies like THRIVE market. When the company Mylan, the supplier of the EpiPen®, a lifesaving medication for people with anaphylactic allergies, raised the price of their product by over 400 percent, consumers started an immediate internet revolution. In a matter of days, it became impossible to ignore the many postings and pleas to make this medication accessible. The media and congressional representatives called out the CEO of the company on its decision. The company retracted the escalated rates and made coupons for the EpiPen and EpiPen Jr available. All voices matter, and we can make a difference.

Today's world is a complicated place. Raising children comes with challenges, sometimes requiring parents to make difficult decisions. It is our hope that the information, strategies, and interventions in this book will serve as a roadmap to help you navigate through the inevitable challenges that come with raising a child and help you to arrive at a desired destination.

Further Resources

Chapter one

Books

Bock, Kenneth, and Cameron Stauth. *Healing the New Childhood Epidemics: Autism, ADHD, Asthma, and Allergies: The Groundbreaking Program for the 4-A Disorders.* New York: Ballantine Books, 2008.

Lambert, Beth, and Victoria Kobliner. *A Compromised Generation: the Epidemic of Chronic Illness in America's Children.* Boulder, CO: Sentient Publications, 2010.

Web Resources

The Marshmallow Experiment: https://www.bing.com/videos/search?q=john+walsh+marshmallow+test&qpvt=john+walsh+marshmallow+test&view=detail&mid=2DB1B71D6CBCCB8245DA2DB1B71D6CBCCB8245DA&FORM=VRDGAR

Chapter two

Books

Doidge, Norman. *The Brain That Changes Itself*. New York: Penguin Books, 2007.

Nemechek, Patrick M., and Jean R. Nemechek. *The Nemechek Protocol™ For Autism and Developmental Disorders: A How-To-Guide for Restoring Neurological Function*. Autonomic Recovery, LLC, 2017.

Emoto, Masaru. *The Hidden Messages in Water*. Hillsboro, OR: Beyond Words Publishing, 2004.

Web Resources

The Hidden Messages in Water: http://www.masaru-emoto.net/english/water-crystal.html

Chapter three

Books

Moore, Polly. *The Natural Baby Sleep Solution: Use Your Child's Internal Sleep Rhythms for Better Nights and Naps*. New York: Workman Publishing, 2016.

Murkoff, Heidi Eisenberg., and Sharon Mazel. *What to Expect the First Year*. New York: Simon & Schuster, 2004. (There are other books in this series for different ages and stages.)

Murkoff, Heidi Eisenberg., and Sharon Mazel. *What to Expect When You're Expecting*. New York: Workman Publishing, 2016.

Chapter four

Books

Dorfman, Kelly. *Cure Your Child with Food: The Hidden Connection between Nutrition and Childhood Ailments*. New York: Workman Publishing, 2013.

Geary, Natalie, and Oz Garcia. *The Food Cure for Kids: A Nutritional Approach to Your Child's Wellness*. Guilford, CT: Lyons Press, 2010.

McDermott, Barbara. *Food BS: Peace, Truth, Science*. Fort Myers Beach, FL: SHIFT Formula, 2017.

O'Brien, Robyn. *The Unhealthy Truth*. New York: Broadway Books, 2009.

Scott, Trudy. *The Anti-Anxiety Food Solution: How the Foods You Eat Can Help You Calm Your Anxious Mind, Improve Your Mood, & End Cravings*. New Harbinger Publications, 2011.

Web Resources

Weston A. Price Foundation (information on nutrition): https://www.westona-price.org/

Free information on food allergies: http://www.allergykids.com

Time Magazine article on GMOs (2015): http://time.com/3840073/gmo-food-charts/

More info on GMOs: https://www.nongmoproject.org/

Decipher serving sizes for your child customized by age, gender, activity level: http://www.buildhealthykids.com/servingsizes.html

"Think Dirty" app: you can download this app onto your phone. It allows you to scan an item's barcode and it will give you an easy-to-read report on the product's ingredients.

https://thrivemarket.com/

Chapter five

Books

Conner, Bobbi. *Unplugged Play: No Batteries, No Plugs, Pure Fun.* New York: Workman Publishing, 2007.

Louv, Richard. *Last Child in the Woods: Saving Our Children from Nature-Deficit Disorder.* Chapel Hill, NC: Algonquin Books, 2008.

Healy, Jane M. *Endangered Minds: Why Children Don't Think—and What We Can Do about It.* New York: Simon & Schuster, 1999.

Hirsch-Pasek, Kathy, and Roberta Michnick Golinkoff. *Einstein Never Used Flashcards: How Our Children Really Learn—and Why They Need to Play More and Memorize Less.* Emmaus, PA: Rodale Books, 2003.

Web Resources

Play and Playground Encyclopedia: https://www.pgpedia.com/h/kathy-hirsh-pasek

Chapter six

Books

Dunckley, Victoria. *Reset Your Child's Brain: A Four-Week Plan to End Meltdowns, Raise Grades, and Boost Social Skills by Reversing the Effects of Electronic Screen-Time.* Novato, CA: New World Library, 2015.

Kardaras, Nicholas. *Glow Kids: How Screen Addiction Is Hijacking Our Kids—and How to Break the Trance.* New York: St. Martin's Griffin, 2017.

Rowan, Cris. *Virtual Child: The Terrifying Truth about What Technology Is Doing to Children.* Sechelt, Canada: Sunshine Coast Occupational Therapy Inc., 2010.

Twenge, Jean M. *iGen: Why Today's Super-Connected Kids Are Growing up Less Rebellious, More Tolerant, Less Happy—and Completely Unprepared for Adulthood—and What This Means for the Rest of Us)*. New York: Atria Books, 2017.

Web Resources

Hands Free Mama Blog: https://www.handsfreemama.com/2017/12/15/tether-yourself-the-enlightening-talk-parents-arent-having-can-keep-teens-from-a-damaging-drift/

Zone'In Programs Inc.: http://www.zonein.ca/

Safe Sleeves: https://www.energpolarit.com/category.aspx?cid=219

Chapter seven

Books

Hallowell, Edward M. *Crazybusy: Overstretched, Overbooked, and about to Snap! Strategies for Handling Your Fast-Paced Life*. New York: Ballantine Books, 2007

Chapter eight

Books

Borba, Michelle. *Parents Do Make a Difference: How to Raise Kids with Solid Character, Strong Minds, and Caring Hearts*. San Francisco: Jossey-Bass, 1999.

Borba, Michelle. *UnSelfie: Why Empathetic Kids Succeed in Our All-About-Me World*. New York: Touchstone/Simon Schuster, 2016.

Chapman, Gary, and Ross Campbell. *The Five Love Languages of Children*. Chicago: Northfield Publishing, 1997.

Hicks, MaryBeth. *Bringing Up Geeks: Genuine, Enthusiastic, Empowered Kids*. New York: Penguin, 2008.

Leman, Kevin. *Making Children Mind without Losing Yours*. Grand Rapids, MI: Baker Publishing, 2000.

Leman, Kevin. *The Birth Order Book: Why You Are the Way You Are*. Grand Rapids, MI: Revell, 2009.

Levine, Madeline. *The Price of Privilege*. New York: HarperCollins, 2006.

Lythcott-Haims, Judith. *How to Raise an Adult*. New York: St. Martin's Press, 2015.

Marano, Hara Estroff. *A Nation of Wimps: The High Cost of Invasive Parenting*. New York: Broadway Books, 2008.

Mogul, Wendy. *The Blessing of a Skinned Knee*. New York: Scribner, 2001.

Phelan, Thomas. *1-2-3 Magic: Effective Discipline for Children 2–12*. Glen Ellyn, IL: Child Management, 2003.

Taffel, Ron. *Childhood Unbound: Saving Our Kids' Best Selves—Confident Parenting in a World of Change*. New York: Simon and Schuster.

Vannoy, Steven. *The Ten Greatest Gifts I Give My Children: Parenting from the Heart*. New York: Simon and Schuster, 1994.

Walsh, David. *No: Why Kids—of All Ages—Need to Hear It and Ways Parents Can Say It*. New York: Free Press, 2007.

Chapter nine

Books

Barrickman, Lisa. *A Case for Kindness: 40 Ways to Love and Inspire Others*. Worthy Publishing Group, 2017.

Jones, Charlotte Foltz. *Mistakes That Worked: 40 Familiar Inventions and How They Came to Be*. New York: Delacorte Press, 1991.

Madigan, Jean Blaydes. *Thinking on Your Feet—200 Activities That Move Kids to Learn*. Huger, SC: Action Based Learning, LLC: 2000.

Thompson, Susan. *Handy Learning: Activities for Hand Development and Curriculum Enhancement*. Flower Mound, TX: Handy Learning Seminars, Inc., 2008.

Web Resources

Conflict Resolution: https://youthlight.com/search.php?p=peace+walk

How Does Your Engine Run? The Alert Program: www.alertprogram.com/?s=
how+does+your+engine+run?

Pipsqueak Markers: These can be found in most stores that carry school supplies. Here is an example of what they look like: https://www.amazon.com/
Crayola-Pip-Squeaks-Washable-Markers-Perfect/dp/B003HGGPM6

Crayon Rocks: These can be found in most stores that carry school supplies.
Here is an example of what they look like: https://www.amazon.com/Crayon-
Rocks-Colors-Red-Velvet/dp/B002EODQBA/ref=sr_1_5?ie=UTF8&qid=15
35547870&sr=8-5&keywords=crayons+rocks&dpID=41ZkYUQrP4L&pre
ST=_SX300_QL70_&dpSrc=srch

Reading Aids

EZC Reader Strips for young readers: https://www.reallygoodstuff.com/
return-sweep-ezc-reader/p/121824/?green=5FC43EE3-2269-5B0B-A731-
1146AA2C493B&MBTZ=mb_catalog&MBP=prod

EZC Reader Strips for older readers: https://www.reallygoodstuff.com/
ezc-reader-strips/p/143538/?green=5FC43EE3-2269-5B0B-A731-
1146AA2C493B&MBTZ=mb_catalog&MBP=prod

Shoe-Tying Tips

http://mamaot.com/teach-kids-tie-shoes-tips-tricks-modifications/

http://www.efficientlifeskills.com/how-i-taught-my-6-year-old-to-tie-shoes-in-
5-minutes/

https://therapyfunzone.net/blog/teaching-shoe-tying-tips-and-tricks/

Superbrain Yoga

http://www.collective-evolution.com/2015/09/06/superbrain-yoga-3-minutes-
that-maximize-brain-power/

http://www.stepbystep.com/how-to-do-superbrain-yoga-34188/

Weighted Blankets and Animals

https://www.therapyshoppe.com/category/P269-dolphin-wrap-weighted-animals-pressure-pets-sensory-toys

http://www.mosaicweightedblankets.com/benefits/ or http://www.sensory-processing-disorder.com/

Chapter ten

Books

Cook, Sandra K. *The Dyslexia Help Handbook for Parents: Your Guide to Overcoming Dyslexia Including Tools You Can Use for Learning Empowerment.* Publisher Not Identified, 2014.

Kranowitz, Carol Stock. *The Out-of-Sync Child: Recognizing and Coping with Sensory Processing Disorder.* Paradise, CA: Paw Prints, 2011.

Kranowitz, Carol Stock., and T. J. Wylie. *The Goodenoughs Get in Sync: 5 Family Members Overcome Their Special Sensory Issues.* Arlington, TX: Sensory World, 2010.

Moize, Jean, and Cindy Hess. *Action Based Learning: Primary Lab Manual.* Huger, SC: Kidsfit Publishing, 2018.

Web Resources

Holistic Health International: http://www.holisticheal.com/books-and-dvds/free-online-videos

Able Kids Foundation: http://www.ablekidsfoundation.org/

Orton Gillingham Reading Approach: https://www.ortonacademy.org/resources/what-is-the-orton-gillingham-approach/

Wilson Reading: https://www.wilsonlanguage.com/programs/wilson-reading-system/

Action Based Learning

http://www.youthfit.com/ABL

http://actionbasedlearning.3dcartstores.com/All-Lab-Stations_c_13.html

www.abllab.com

Acupuncture/Acupressure: http://www.acupressure.com

Chiropractic/NRT
http://b2hc.com/

https://www.mcgaurnfamilychiro.com/

Emotional Freedom Technique:
www.thetappingsolution.com

www.eftuniverse.com

https://www.thetappingpractice.com

www.createglobalhealing.org

www.thetappingsolutionfoundation.com

www.jesselewischooselove.org

Epigenetics: http://www.superconsciousness.com/topics/science/interview-dr-bruce-lipton

Eye Movement Desensitization and Reprocessing (EMDR)
http://www.emdr.com/

http://emdria.site-ym.com/?page=Neurobiological

FM Systems
https://classroom.synonym.com/fm-listening-systems-classroom-7866485.html

FastForWord®
http://www.scilearn.com

http://www.scilearn.com/for-parents/work-with-a-provider/search-for-a-provider

Forbrain®: https://www.forbrain.com/

Homeopathy
https://www.homeopathyusa.org/

http://drpeterprociuk.com/drpeterprociuk.com/home.html

Integrative Medicine: https://www.aihm.org

Interactive Metronome®
http://www.interactivemetronome.com

https://www.youtube.com/watch?v=H8d4pAQo9T4

https://www.youtube.com/watch?v=kLOXiDvjwnY

Lindamood Bell Programs
http://lindamoodbell.com/our-approach

https://magazine.washington.edu/feature/dyslexia/

Methylation Pathways and Nutrigenomics: http://www.holistichealth.com

Neuro Emotional Technique (NET)
www.netmindbody.com

www.onefoundation.org

http://www.christinehannafin.com

Neurofeedback
http://www.aboutneurofeedback.com/neurofeedback-info-center/faq/
how-does-neurofeedback-work/what-is-neurofeedback/

http://www.brandywinevalleycc.com

Sensory Integration
http://www.sensory-processing-disorder.com/ https://www.nationalautismresourc-
es.com/the-wilbarger-protocol-brushing-therapy-for-sensory-integration/

http://www.atotalapproach.com

Tomatis®: http://www.tomatis.com/en/tomatis-method/research-and-results/
psychological-disorders.html

Vision Therapy
http://www.drchayaherzberg.com

www.eyecanlearn.com

www.Irlen.com

Conclusion

Web Resources

Environmental Working Group, watchdog group for consumer safety: https://www.ewg.org

Documenting Hope: https://documentinghope.com

Image Credits

Endnotes

Introduction

1   Allen Frances, "10,000 Young Toddlers Are on Stimulant Drugs for ADHD," *Huffington Post*, May 17, 2014, https://www.huffingtonpost.com/allen-frances/adhd-toddler-diagnosis_b_5343766.html.

2   Tom Huddleston Jr., "Sean Parker Wonders What Facebook Is 'Doing to Our Children's Brains,'" *Fortune*, November 9, 2017, fortune.com/2017/11/09/sean-parker-facebook-childrens-brains/.

3   David Meyer, "Facebook Is 'Ripping Apart' Society, Former Executive Warns." *Fortune*, December 12, 2017, fortune.com/2017/12/12/chamath-palihapitiya-facebook-society/.

Chapter one

1   Pennsylvania Department of Education, Education Budget, http://www.education.pa.gov/teachers%20-%20administrators/school%20finances/education%20budget/pages/default.aspx.

2   Kenneth Bock, Cameron Stauth, and Korri Fink, *Healing the New Childhood Epidemics: Autism, ADHD, Asthma, and Allergies: The Groundbreaking Program for the 4-A Disorders* (New York: Ballantine, 2008), 17.

3   Bock, Stauth, and Fink, *Healing the New Childhood Epidemics*, 17.

4   "Medical and Scientific Literature." Documenting Hope, September 15, 2017.

5   "Childhood Cancers," National Cancer Institute, http://www.cancer.gov/research/progress/snapshots/pediatric.

6   Bock, Stauth, and Fink, *Healing the New Childhood Epidemics*, 173.

7   Bock, Stauth, and Fink, *Healing the New Childhood Epidemics*, 173.

8   Bock, Stauth, and Fink, *Healing the New Childhood Epidemics*, 174.

9   http://www.diabetesforecast.org/2012/nov/more-kids-than ever-have-type-2-diabetes.html

10   Beth Lambert and Victoria Kobliner, *A Compromised Generation: The Epidemic of Chronic Illness in America's Children* (Boulder, CO: Sentient Publications, 2010), 14.

11   "Any Anxiety Disorder Among Children," National Institute of Mental Health, U.S. Department of Health and Human Services, September 15, 2017, https://www.nimh.nih.gov/health/statistics/any-anxiety-disorder.shtml.

12   Centers for Disease Control and Prevention, "Child Abuse and Neglect Cost the United States $124 billion," Press release, February 1, 2012, https://www.cdc.gov/media/releases/2012/p0201_child_abuse.html.

13   Robert F. Anda and Vincent Felitti, "Adverse Childhood Experiences and Their Relationship to Adult Well-being and Disease: Turning Gold into Lead," The National Council webinar, August 27, 2012, https://www.thenationalcouncil.org/wp-content/uploads/2012/11/Natl-Council-Webinar-8-2012.pdf.

14   "The ACE Score," The Adverse Childhood Experiences Study: A Springboard to Hope, www.acestudy.org/the-ace-score.html.

15   Donna Jackson Nakazawa, "Childhood Trauma Leads to Lifelong Chronic Illness—So Why Isn't the Medical Community Helping Patients?" *Huffington Post*, July 29, 2016, https://www.huffingtonpost.com/donna-jackson-nakazawa/childhood-trauma-leads-to_b_11154082.html.

16   James W. Prescott, "America's Lost Dream," Association for Prenatal and Pernatal Psychology and Health, 10th International Congress, Institute of Humanistic Science, http://www.violence.de/prescott/appp/ald.pdf.

17   Jean M. Twenge, Thomas E. Joiner, Megan L. Rogers, et al., "Increases in Depressive Symptoms, Suicide-Related Outcomes, and Suicide Rates Among U.S. Adolescents After 2010 and Links to Increased New Media Screen Time," *Clinical Psychological Science* 6 (2018), http://journals.sagepub.com/doi/full/10.1177/2167702617723376.

18   Jean Twenge, "With Teen Mental Health Deteriorating over Five Years, There's a Likely Culprit," *The Conversation*, November 14, 2017, https://theconversation.com/with-teen-mental-health-deteriorating-over-five-years-theres-a-likely-culprit-86996.

19   Centers for Disease Control and Prevention, Youth Risk Behavior and Surveillance System, https://www.cdc.gov/healthyyouth/data/yrbs/index.htm.

20   Sally S. Curtin, Margaret Warner, and Holly Hedegaard, "Increase in Suicide in the United States, 1999–2014," NCHS Data Brief, No. 241, April 2016, https://www.cdc.gov/nchs/products/databriefs/db241.htm.

21   Twenge, Joiner, and Rogers, "Increases in Depressive Symptoms."

22   Bock, Stauth, and Fink, *Healing the New Childhood Epidemics* p. 17

23   National Center for Education Statistics, "Fast Facts: Students with Disabilities," 2018, https://nces.ed.gov/fastfacts/display.asp?id=64.

24 National Center for Health Statistics, *Health, United States, 2014: With Special Feature on Adults Aged 55–64*, Hyattsville, MD, 2015,

http://www.cdc.gov/nchs/data/hus/hus14.pdf#glance.

25 LaJeana D. Howie, Patricia N. Pastor, and Susan L. Lukacs, "Use of Medication Prescribed for Emotional or Behavioral Difficulties among Children Aged 6–17 Years in the United States, 2011–2012," NCHS Data Brief, No. 148, April 2014, https://www.cdc.gov/nchs/data/databriefs/db148.pdf.

26 http://pediatrics.aappublications.org/content/pediatrics/early/2012/06/13/peds.2011-2879.full.pdf

27 Andres Martin and Douglas Leslie, "Trends in Psychotropic Medication Costs for Children and Adolescents, 1997–2000," *Archives of Pediatric and Adolescent Medicine* 157 (2003): 997–1004, https://pdfs.semanticscholar.org/0fdd/f506cceba3652bff4fada32ffa6d02e419b8.pdf.

28 Bock, Stauth, and Fink, *Healing the New Childhood Epidemics*. p 337

29 Martin and Leslie, "Trends in Psychotropic Medication Costs."

30 A. Pawlowski, "'That's Nuts': 10,000 Toddlers Get Drugs for ADHD." *TODAY.com*, May 19, 2014.

31 Alan Schwarz, "The Selling of Attention Deficit Disorder," *New York Times*, December 14, 2013, http://www.nytimes.com/2013/12/15/health/the-selling-of-attention-deficit-disorder.html?pagewanted=all.

32 Mark Hyman, *The UltraMind Solution: Companion Guide*, UtraWellness, LLC, http://drhyman.com/downloads/UltraMindCompanionGuide.pdf.

33 National Center for Education Statistics, "The NCES Fast Facts Tool Provides Quick Answers to Many Education Questions," September 15, 2017.

34 R. Giuliani and G. Pierangelo, "Prevalence of Learning Disabilities," *Education.com*, July 20, 2010, http://www.education.com/reference/article/prevalence-learning-disabilities/.

35 Bock, Stauth, and Fink, *Healing the New Childhood Epidemics, 175.*

36 Nirvi Shah, "More Students Receiving Accommodations During ACT, SAT," *Education Week*—On Special Education, May 14, 2012, http://blogs.edweek.org/edweek/speced/2012/05/more_students_receiving_accomm.html

37 Shah, "More Students Receiving Accommodations During ACT, SAT."

38 National Center for Education Statistics, "Fast Facts: Students with Disabilities," 2018, https://nces.ed.gov/fastfacts/display.asp?id=64.

39 Centers for Disease Control and Prevention, "Key Findings: Trends in the Prevalence of Developmental Disabilities in U.S. Children, 1997–2008," February 12, 2015, https://www.cdc.gov/ncbddd/developmentaldisabilities/features/birthdefects-dd-keyfindings.html.

40 National Center for Education Statistics, "Fast Facts: Students with Disabilities," 2018, https://nces.ed.gov/fastfacts/display.asp?id=64.

41 Maria Konnikova, "The Struggles of a Psychologist Studying Self-Control," *The New Yorker*, October 9, 2014, http://www.newyorker.com/science/maria-konnikova/struggles-psychologist-studying-self-control.

42 Jill Anderson, "Pathways to Prosperity Releases New Reports," Harvard Graduate School of Education, July 1, 2014, https://www.gse.harvard.edu/news/14/07/pathways-prosperity-releases-new-reports.

43 Lou Carlozo, "Why College Students Stop Short of a Degree," *Reuters*, March 27, 2012, https://www.reuters.com/article/us-attn-andrea-education-dropouts/why-college-students-stop-short-of-a-degree-idUSBRE82Q0Y120120327.

44 Ted Dintersmith and Tony Wagner, "America Desperately Needs to Redefine 'College and Career Ready,'" *MarketWatch*, August 31, 2016, https://www.marketwatch.com/story/america-desperately-needs-to-redefine-college-and-career-ready-2016-08-05.

Chapter two

1 "Medical Definition of Neuroplasticity," MedicineNet, www.medicinenet.com/script/main/art.asp?articlekey=40362.

2 "Brain and Nervous System," Edited by Steven Dowshen, KidsHealth, The Nemours Foundation, July 2015, kidshealth.org/en/parents/brain-nervous-system.html#.

3 Norman Doidge, *The Brain That Changes Itself: Stories of Personal Triumph from the Frontiers of Brain Science* (New York: Penguin Books, 2007), 53–54.

4 Doidge, *The Brain That Changes Itself*.

5 "Upstairs and Downstairs Brain," Momentous Institute, November 12, 2014, http://momentousinstitute.org/blog/upstairs-and-downstairs-brain.

6 Susan L. Nasr, "How Brain Mapping Works," HowStuffWorks Science, August 14, 2008, https://science.howstuffworks.com/life/inside-the-mind/human-brain/brain-mapping.htm.

7 "Broca's Area Is the Brain's Scriptwriter, Shaping Speech, Study Finds," Johns Hopkins Medicine, Press Release, February 17, 2015, https://www.hopkinsmedicine.org/news/media/releases/brocas_area_is_the_brains_scriptwriter_shaping_speech_study_finds.

8 Susan Scutti, "Dyslexia 'Seen' In Brain Scans of Kindergartners: Earlier Learning Interventions May Be Possible," *Medical Daily*, August 14, 2013, www.medicaldaily.com/dyslexia-seen-brain-scans-kindergartners-earlier-learning-interventions-may-be-possible-251307.

9 Regina Bailey. "Afraid? Blame Your Amygdala." ThoughtCo., https://www.thoughtco.com/amygdala-anatomy-373211.

10 "SPECT Scan," Mayo Clinic, December 23, 2016, https://www.mayoclinic.org/tests-procedures/spect-scan/home/ovc-20303153.

11 https://en.wikipedia.org/wiki/Limbic_system

12 Doidge, *The Brain That Changes Itself*, 59.

13 "Microglia: The Constant Gardeners." *Nature News*, May 30, 2012, https://www.nature.com/news/microglia-the-constant-gardeners-1.10732.

14 Doidge, *The Brain That Changes Itself*, 47.

15 Doidge, *The Brain That Changes Itself*, 68.

16 "Otto Loewi–Biographical," Nobelprize.org, https://www.nobelprize.org/nobel_prizes/medicine/laureates/1936/loewi-bio.html.

17 Annamarya Scaccia, "Serotonin: Functions, Side Effects, and More," Healthline, May 18, 2017, www.healthline.com/health/mental-health/serotonin#mental-health.

18 Healthline Editorial Team, "7 Foods That Could Boost Your Serotonin," Healthline, July 10, 2017, www.healthline.com/health/healthy-sleep/foods-that-could-boost-your-serotonin?m=2.

19 Christopher Heffner, "Chapter 2: Section 2: Neurotransmitters." AllPsych, allpsych.com/psychology101/neurotransmitters/.

20 Elizabeth Renter, "How to Increase Dopamine Levels: Foods to Eat and What to Do." Natural Society, February 19, 2013, naturalsociety.com/how-to-increase-dopamine-levels-foods/.

21 "Integrative Psychiatry," Integrative Psychiatry: Lab Testing, Neurotransmitters & Mental Health Supplements, September 17, 2017.

22 Doidge, *The Brain That Changes Itself*, 69.

23 Doidge, *The Brain That Changes Itself*, 71–72.

24 Doidge, *The Brain That Changes Itself*, 73.

25 Gabrielle Emanuel, "Millions Have Dyslexia, Few Understand It," NPR, November 28, 2016, https://www.npr.org/sections/ed/2016/11/28/502601662/millions-have-dyslexia-few-understand-it.

26 Carl Bianco, "How Your Heart Works," HowStuffWorks, April 1, 2000, http://health.howstuffworks.com/human-body/systems/circulatory/heart4.htm.

27 Robert O. Becker, "Modern Bioelectromagnetics and Functions of the Central Nervous System," *ISSSEEM* 3 (1992), http://journals.sfu.ca/seemj/index.php/seemj/article/view/145.

28 Masaru Emoto, *The Hidden Messages in Water* (Hillsboro, OR: Beyond Words Publishing, 2004), xxiv.

29 Emoto, *The Hidden Messages in Water*, xv.

30 Brent Lambert, "Harvard Unveils MRI Study Proving Meditation Literally Rebuilds The Brain's Gray Matter In 8 Weeks," *FEELguide*. November 19, 2014, https://www.feelguide.com/2014/11/19/harvard-unveils-mri-study-proving-meditation-literally-rebuilds-the-brains-gray-matter-in-8-weeks/.

31 "Three More Health Benefits of Being beside the Sea." Daily Mail Online. Associated Newspapers, 15 Nov. 2002. Web. 19 Sept. 2017.

Chapter three

1   Sue Goode, Martha Diefendorf, and Siobhan Colgan, "The Importance of Early Intervention for Infants and Toddlers with Disabilities and Their Families," NEATAC, July 2011, http://www.nectac.org/~pdfs/pubs/importanceofearlyintervention.pdf.

2   "Ages 0–2: Developmental Overview." ParentFurther, March 26, 2015, https://www.parentfurther.com/content/ages-0-2-developmental-overview.

3   District of Columbia Public Schools, "Child Developmental Milestones," 2011, http://aapdc.org/wp-content/uploads/2014/01/Early-Stages-Milestones-EN-2011.pdf.

4   Centers for Disease Control and Prevention, "Important Milestones: Your Baby by Four Months," October 25, 2017, https://www.cdc.gov/ncbddd/actearly/milestones/milestones-4mo.html.

5   "Ages 3–5: Developmental Overview," ParentFurther, March 26, 2015, https://www.parentfurther.com/content/ages-3-5-developmental-overview.

6   "Ages 6–6: Developmental Overview," ParentFurther, March 26, 2015, https://www.parentfurther.com/content/ages-6-9-developmental-overview

7   "Ages 10–14: Developmental Overview," ParentFurther, March 26, 2015, https://www.parentfurther.com/content/ages-10-14-developmental-overview.

8   Mette Morell, "Neuroplasticity Psychology: Synaptic Pruning," SlideShare, https://www.slideshare.net/mettemorell/neuroplasticity-psychology-ib.

9   Robin Marantz Henig, "What Is It About 20-Somethings?" *New York Times Magazine*, August 18, 2010, http://www.nytimes.com/2010/08/22/magazine/22Adulthood-t.html?pagewanted=all.

10   "Ages 10–14: Developmental Milestones," ParentFurther, May 25, 2017, https://www.parentfurther.com/content/ages-10-14-developmental-overview.

11   Daniel J. Siegel, "Pruning, Myelination, and the Remodeling Adolescent Brain," Psychology Today, February 4, 2014, https://www.psychologytoday.com/blog/inspire-rewire/201402/pruning-myelination-and-the-remodeling-adolescent-brain.

12   "Sleep Drive and Your Body Clock," National Sleep Foundation, sleepfoundation.org/sleep-topics/sleep-drive-and-your-body-clock/page/0/1.

13   Boston Children's Hospital, ""Later Start Times Better for High School Students: Poor Self-Regulation in Teens Linked to Circadian Rhythms: Findings Support Later Start Times for Middle Schools and High Schools," ScienceDaily, November 3, 2016, www.sciencedaily.com/releases/2016/11/161103130300.htm.

14   "Ages 15–18: Developmental Overview," ParentFurther, May 25, 2017, https://www.parentfurther.com/content/ages-15-18-developmental-overview.

15   Cornelius K. Donat, Gregory Scott, Steve M. Gentleman, and Magdalena Sastre, "Microglial Activation in Traumatic Brain Injury," *Frontiers in Aging Neuroscience* 9 (2017): 208, https://www.ncbi.nlm.nih.gov/pmc/articles/PMC5487478/.

16   "Autonomic Recover and Inflammation," Nemechek Autonomic Medicine, https://www.nemechekconsultativemedicine.com/inflammation/.

Chapter four

1   Natalie Geary and Oz Garcia, *The Food Cure for Kids: A Nutritional Approach to Your Child's Wellness* (Guilford, CT: Lyons Press, 2010), 15.

2   Geary and Garcia, *The Food Cure for Kids*, 84–87.

3   Silvia Slazenger, "Inflammatory Symptoms, Immune System and Food Intolerance: One Cause—Many Symptoms," Cell Science Systems, July 29, 2015, https://cellsciencesystems.com/education/research/inflammatory-symptoms-immune-system-and-food-intolerance-one-cause-many-symptoms/.

4   "Gut Inflammation and Your Brain," davidperlmutter MD, https://www.drperlmutter.com/gut-inflammation-affects-brain/.

5   Rachel Labidos, "Could the Root Cause of Depression Be in Your Gut—and Not Your Brain?" Well + Good, June 12, 2016, https://www.wellandgood.com/good-advice/depression-gut-inflammation-connection-kelly-brogan/.

6   Nemechek, *The Nemechek Protocol For Autism and Developmental Delays.*

7   "The Nutrition Deficit Disorder (NDD) Book by Dr. Sears," Bynature.ca, 2012, http://www.bynature.ca/the-nutrition-deficit-disorder-book-by-dr-sears.html.

8   Rebecca Harrington, "Does Artificial Food Coloring Contribute to ADHD in Children?" *Scientific American*, April 27, 2015, https://www.scientificamerican.com/article/does-artificial-food-coloring-contribute-to-adhd-in-children/.

9   Courtney Williams, "Calming Our Children: An Examination of the Fein-gold Diet," Health Psychology Home Page, Vanderbilt University, http://healthpsych.psy.vanderbilt.edu/2008/FeingoldDiet.htm.

10   "Aspartame: The Most Dangerous Substance on the Market," Mercola.com, https://articles.mercola.com/sites/articles/archive/2011/11/06/aspartame-most-danger-ous-substance-added-to-food.aspx.

11   Edward Group, "The Health Dangers of Aspartame," Dr. Group's Healthy Living Articles, Global Healing Center, Inc., 2015, https://www.globalhealingcenter.com/natural-health/health-dangers-of-aspartame/.

12   Sylvia Booth Hubbard, "Dangers of Aspartame: What You Need to Know," Newsmax, April 27, 2015, https://www.newsmax.com/Health/Headline/aspartame-sweetener-artificial-Diet-Pepsi/2015/04/27/id/640970/.

13   David A. Kessler, *The End of Overeating: Taking Control of the Insatiable American Appetite* (Emmaus, PA: Rodale, 2010).

14   Hilary Parker, "A Sweet Problem: Princeton Researchers Find That High-Fructose Corn Syrup Prompts Considerably More Weight Gain." Princeton University, March 22, 2010, https://www.princeton.edu/main/news/archive/S26/91/22K07/.

15   Sabrina Tavernise, "F.D.A. Makes It Official: BPA Can't Be Used in Baby Bottles and Cups," *New York Times*, July 17, 2012, http://www.nytimes.com/2012/07/18/science/fda-bans-bpa-from-baby-bottles-and-sippy-cups.html.

16 "NTP Finalizes Report on Bisphenol A," National Institute of Environmental Health Sciences, U.S. Department of Health and Human Services, News Release, September 3, 2008, https://www.niehs.nih.gov/news/newsroom/releases/2008/september03/.

17 Elizabeth Kolbert, "A Warning by Key Researcher on Risks of BPA in Our Lives," YaleEnvironment 360, November 24, 2010, https://e360.yale.edu/feature/a_warning_by_key_researcher_on_risks_of_bpa_in_our_lives/2344/.

18 Roddy Scheer and Doug Moss, "Why Are Trace Chemicals Showing Up in Umbilical Cord Blood?" *Scientific American*, EarthTalk, https://www.scientificamerican.com/article/chemicals-umbilical-cord-blood/.

19 "Congenital Minamata Disease," Minamata Disease, https//minamatadisease.weebly.com.

20 "Mercury: The Adverse Health Effects of Mercury," University of Minnesota, 2013, http://enhs.umn.edu/current/5103_spring2003/mercury/merchealtheffects.html.

21 U.S. Environmental Protection Agency, Summary of the Toxic Substances Control Act, June 22, 2016, https://www.epa.gov/laws-regulations/summary-toxic-substances-control-act.

22 U.S. Environmental Protection Agency, "The Frank R. Lautenberg Chemical Safety for the 21st Century Act," June 22, 2016, https://www.epa.gov/assessing-and-managing-chemicals-under-tsca/frank-r-lautenberg-chemical-safety-21st-century-act.

23 Michael Pollan, "Playing God in the Garden," *New York Times Magazine*, October 25, 1998, https://www.nytimes.com/1998/10/25/magazine/playing-god-in-the-garden.html.

24 "MIT Researcher: Glyphosate Herbicide will Cause Half of All Children to Have Autism by 2025," Health Impact News, 2014, https://healthimpactnews.com/2014/mit-researcher-glyphosate-herbicide-will-cause-half-of-all-children-to-have-autism-by-2025/.

25 Monika Krüger, Philipp Schledorn, Wieland Schrödl, Hans-Wolfgang Hoppe, Walburga Lutz, and Awad A. Shehata, "Detection of Glyphosate Residues in Animals and Humans," *Journal of Environmental & Analytical Toxicology* 4 (2014): 2.

26 "MIT Researcher: Glyphosate Herbicide Will Cause Half of All Children to Have Autism by 2025," Health Impact News.

27 "MIT Researcher: Glyphosate Herbicide Will Cause Half of All Children to Have Autism by 2025," Health Impact News.

28 Susan Scutti, "Autism Rates to Increase by 2025? Glyphosate Herbicide May Be Responsible for Future Half of Children with Autism," *Medical Daily*, January 5, 2015, https://www.medicaldaily.com/autism-rates-increase-2025-glyphosate-herbicide-may-be-responsible-future-half-316388.

29 Jörgen Magnér, Petra Wallberg, Jasmin Sandberg, and Anna Palm Cousins, "Human exposure to pesticides from food A pilot study," NR U 5080, January 2015, https://www.coop.se/contentassets/dc9bd9f95773402997e4aca0c11b8274/coop-ekoefekten_rapport_eng.pdf.

30 David Gutierrez, "Eating Organic Foods Reduces Pesticide Exposure by Nearly 90% After Just One Week," Natural News, May 6, 2014, https://www.natural-news.com/045006_organic_foods_pesticide_exposure_phthalates.html.

31 Deanna Minich, "Why You Should Break a Sweat Every Day," *Huffington Post*, November 30, 2016, https://www.huffingtonpost.com/deanna-minich-phd/4-reasons-to-break-a-swea_b_13305850.html.

32 Julie Revelant, "10 Ways to Rid Your Body of Toxic Chemicals," Fox News Health, June 9, 2014, http://www.foxnews.com/health/2014/06/09/10-ways-to-rid-your-body-toxic-chemicals.html.

33 Mary Mullen and Jo Ellen Shield, "Water: How Much Do Kids Need?" Eat Right, May 2, 2017, http://www.eatright.org/resource/fitness/sports-and-performance/hydrate-right/water-go-with-the-flow.

34 Neil Osterweil, "The Benefits of Protein," WebMD, https://www.webmd.com/men/features/benefits-protein#1.

35 "Good Protein Sources," WebMD, https://www.webmd.com/fitness-exercise/guide/good-protein-sources.

36 Jessie Szalay, "What Are Carbohydrates?" Live Science, July 14, 2017, https://www.livescience.com/51976-carbohydrates.html.

37 "What Are Healthy Simple Carbohydrates?" SFGate, http://healthyeating.sfgate.com/healthy-simple-carbohydrates-6348.html.

38 Szalay, "What Are Carbohydrates."

39 "Carbohydrates: Complex Carbs vs. Simple Carbs," Physicians Committee for Responsible Medicine, http://www.nutritionmd.org/nutrition_tips/nutrition_tips_understand_foods/carbs_versus.html.

40 Katherine Sellgrem, "Why Spending Time Outdoors Could Help Your Child's Eyesight," BBC News, December 28, 2017, http://www.bbc.com/news/health-42238691.

41 Geary and Garcia, *The Food Cure for Kids*, 124–127.

42 Geary and Garcia, *The Food Cure for Kids*, 127, 132.

43 Sarah-Jane Bedwell and Amy Marturana, "19 Healthy Fats and High-Fat Foods You Should Be Eating," *Self*, December 27, 2016, https://www.self.com/story/9-high-fat-foods-actually-good-for-you.

44 "Memo to Pediatricians: Screen All Kids for Vitamin D Deficiency, Test Those at High Risk," Johns Hopkins Medicine, February 22, 2012, https://www.hopkinsmedicine.org/news/media/releases/memo_to_pediatricians_screen_all_kids_for_vitamin_d_deficiency_test_those_at_high_risk.

45 "7 Signs and Symptoms You May Have a Vitamin D Deficiency," Mercola.com, May 28, 2014, http://articles.mercola.com/sites/articles/archive/2014/05/28/vitamin-d-deficiency-signs-symptoms.aspx.

46 Paul Fassa, "16 Magnesium Deficiency Symptoms—Signs of Low Magnesium Levels," Natural Society, April 1, 2013, http://naturalsociety.com/16-magnesium-deficiency-symptoms-signs-low-levels/.

47 "Iron-Deficiency Anemia," KidsHealth from Nemours, 2014, http://kidshealth.org/en/parents/ida.html.

48 Vincent Pernell, "B Vitamins," www.drpernell.com/b vitamins.htm.

49 Pernell, "B Vitamins."

50 Joseph Nordqvist. "Zinc: Health Benefits and Warnings," *Medical News Today*, December 5, 2017, https://www.medicalnewstoday.com/articles/263176.php.

51 Geary and Garcia, *The Food Cure for Kids*, 77.

52 Geary and Garcia, *The Food Cure for Kids*, 185.

53 "Debunking The Salt Myth: Add This Seasoning to Food Daily," Mercola.com, September 20, 2011, http://articles.mercola.com/sites/articles/archive/2011/09/20/salt-myth.aspx.

54 Sonya Lunder, "EWG's 2017 Shopper's Guide to Pesticides in Produce," EWG, April 10, 2018, https://www.ewg.org/foodnews/summary.php.

55 Arti Patel, "Top Dirty Dozen and Clean 15 Foods," *Huffington Post*, April 30, 2014, https://www.huffingtonpost.ca/2014/04/30/top-dirty-dozen-and-clean_n_5242343.html.

Chapter five

1 Rachel E. White, "The Power of Play: A Research Summary on Play and Learning," Minnesota Children's Museum, July 15, 2016, http://www.childrensmuseums.org/images/MCMResearchSummary.pdf.

2 White, "The Power of Play."

3 Emily Woodbury and Charity Nebbe, "Playgrounds and the Importance of Play," Iowa Public Radio, July 12, 2016, http://iowapublicradio.org/post/playgrounds-and-importance-play.

4 "What Hiking Does To The Brain Is Pretty Amazing," Wimp.com, April 11, 2016, http://www.wimp.com/what-hiking-does-to-the-brain-is-pretty-amazing/.

5 *Where Do the Children Play?* [documentary film], University of Michigan Press, 2008, https://www.press.umich.edu/360473/where_do_the_children_play.

6 Alex Spiegel, "Old-Fashioned Play Builds Serious Skills," NPR, February 21, 2008, http://www.npr.org/templates/story/story.php?storyId=19212514.

7 Spiegel, "Old-Fashioned Play Builds Serious Skills."

8 Peter Gray, "The Decline of Play and Rise in Children's Mental Disorders," Psychology Today, January 26, 2010, https://www.psychologytoday.com/blog/freedom-learn/201001/the-decline-play-and-rise-in-childrens-mental-disorders.

9 "Olweus Bullying Prevention Program, Clemson University," 2013, http://www.clemson.edu/olweus/about.html.

10 "Social Emotional Learning Toolkits—SEL Toolkits," Thom Stecher and Associates, 2015, http://www.seltoolkits.com/index.php/social-emotional-learning-toolkits.html.

11 Susan Thompson, *Handy Learning: Activities for Hand Development and Curriculum Enhancement* (Flower Mound, TX: Handy Learning Seminars, Inc., 2008), 7.

12 Valerie Strauss, "Why So Many Kids Can't Sit Still in School Today," *The Washington Post*, July 8, 2014, https://www.washingtonpost.com/news/answer-sheet/wp/2014/07/08/why-so-many-kids-cant-sit-still-in-school-today/.

13 Strauss, "Why So Many Kids Can't Sit Still in School Today."

14 Jane M. Healy, *Endangered Minds: Why Children Don't Think—and What We Can Do About It* (New York: Simon and Schuster, 1990), 68.

15 Thompson, *Handy Learning*, 7–12.

16 "Play." Definition by Bing.com. https://www.bing.com/search?q=What%20does%20play%20mean&pc=cosp&ptag=C1N0006D010114A316A5D3C6E&form=CONBDF&conlogo=CT3210127.

17 Maria Konnikova, "The Struggles of a Psychologist Studying Self-Control," *The New Yorker*, October 9, 2014, http://www.newyorker.com/science/maria-konnikova/struggles-psychologist-studying-self-control.

18 Thompson, *Handy Learning*, 7–17.

19 "The Role of Mirror Neurons in Human Behavior," *US News*, August 3, 2011, http://www.usnews.com/science/articles/2011/08/03/the-role-of-mirror-neurons-in-human-behavior.

20 Healy, *Endangered Minds*, 95–101.

21 Gwen Dewar, "Can Lego Bricks and Other Construction Toys Boost Your Child's STEM Skills?" Parenting Science, 2013, http://www.parentingscience.com/Lego-bricks-construction-toys-and-STEM-skills.html.

22 Gray, "The Decline of Play and Rise in Children's Mental Disorders."

23 "What Hiking Does to the Brain Is Pretty Amazing," Wimp.com.

24 "Health Benefits," National Wildlife Federation, 2015, http://www.nwf.org/What-We-Do/Kids-and-Nature/Why-Get-Kids-Outside/Health-Benefits.aspx.

25 Katherine Sellgren, "Why Spending Time Outdoors Could Help Your Child's Eyesight," BBC News, December 28, 2017, http://www.bbc.com/news/health-42238691.

26 Thompson, *Handy Learning*, 12.

27 Tim Walker, "The Joyful, Illiterate Kindergartners of Finland," taughtbyfinland.com, October 2, 2015, http://taughtbyfinland.com/the-joyful-illiterate-kindergartners-of-finland/.

28 Valerie Strauss, "How Schools Ruined Recess—and Four Things Needed to Fix It," *The Washington Post*, February 4, 2015, https://www.washingtonpost.com/news/answer-sheet/wp/2015/02/04/how-schools-ruined-recess-and-four-things-needed-to-fix-it/.

29 Elizabeth Licata, "Texas School Triples Recess Time, Sees Positive Results," Scary Mommy, January 9, 2016, http://www.scarymommy.com/texas-school-triples-recess-time-and-sees-immediate-positive-results-in-kids/.

30 "Peaceful Playgrounds Recess Program Kit," Peaceful Playgrounds, 2015, http://peacefulplaygrounds.com/peaceful-playgrounds-recess-program/.

31 Playfit Education, http://www.playfiteducation.com.

Chapter six

1 Rosemary Black, "1 In 10 Video Gamers May Be Addicted: Study," *NY Daily News*, April 20, 2009, https://www.nydailynews.com/life-style/health/1-10-young-video-game-players-exhibit-addiction-characteristics-parents-article-1.362486.

2 Nicholas Kardaras, "It's 'Digital Heroin': How Screens Turn Kids into Psychotic Junkies," *New York Post*, August 27, 2016, http://nypost.com/2016/08/27/its-digital-heroin-how-screens-turn-kids-into-psychotic-junkies/.

3 Jean Twenge, *iGen Why Today's Super Connected Kids Are Growing Up Less Rebellious, More Tolerant, Less Happy—and Completely Unprepared for Adulthood—and What That Means for the Rest of Us* (New York: Simon and Schuster, 2017), 2.

4 "Selected Research on Screen Time and Children," Campaign for a Commercial-Free Childhood, 2014, http://www.screenfree.org/wp-content/uploads/2014/01/screentimefs.pdf.

5 Jane M. Healy, *Endangered Minds: Why Children Don't Think—and What We Can Do about It* (New York: Simon & Schuster, 1999), 99–102.

6 Victoria L. Dunckley, "Screentime Is Making Kids Moody, Crazy and Lazy," Psychology Today, August 18, 2015, https://www.psychologytoday.com/blog/mental-wealth/201508/screentime-is-making-kids-moody-crazy-and-lazy?utm_sq=fnx7r0cgj4.

7 Victoria L. Dunckley, "Gray Matters: Too Much Screen Time Damages the Brain, Psychology Today, February 27, 2014, https://www.psychologytoday.com/blog/mental-wealth/201402/gray-matters-too-much-screen-time-damages-the-brain

8 Dunckley, "Gray Matters."

9 Abigail Elise, "Too Much Screen Time Is Harming Your Child's Brain: How to Protect Your Family," WBAL, January 30, 2017.

10 Healy, *Endangered Minds*.

11 Kyle Stock, Lance Lambert, and David Ingold, "Smartphones Are Killing Americans, but Nobody's Counting," Bloomberg, October 22, 2017, https://www.msn.com/en-us/news/technology/smartphones-are-killing-americans-but-nobody's-counting/ar-AAtQOp7?li=BBnb7Kz.

12 Dunckley, "Screentime Is Making Kids Moody, Crazy and Lazy."

13 "Selected Research on Screen Time and Children," Campaign for a Commercial-Free Childhood.

14 "Technology Myth and Fact Sheet." Moving to Learn, 2016, http://moving-tolearn.ca/2016/technology-myth-and-fact-sheet.

15 Dunckley, "Screentime Is Making Kids Moody, Crazy and Lazy."

16 Renee Bacher, "The Perils of Smartphones," *AARP Magazine*, August/September 2016, 17.

17 Bacher, "The Perils of Smartphones," 17.

18 Jane Brody, "Screen Addiction Is Taking a Toll on Children," *New York Times*, Well blog, July 6, 2016, http://well.blogs.nytimes.com/2015/07/06/screen-addiction-is-taking-a-toll-on-children/.

19 Greg Hughes and Pauline Chlou, "New Research an Eye Opener on Cause of Myopia," CNN, June 1, 2011, http://www.cnn.com/2011/HEALTH/06/01/myopia.causes/.

20 Damon Beres, "Reading on a Screen before Bed Might Be Killing You," *Huffington Post*, December, 23, 2014, http://www.huffingtonpost.com/2014/12/23/reading-before-bed_n_6372828.html.

21 David Thomas, "Technology Tuesday: Devices Banned for Children under 12," November 18, 2014, http://www.raisingboysandgirls.com/raisingboysandgirls-blog/technology-tuesday-devices-banned-for-children-under-12.

22 "Blue Light Has a Dark Side," Harvard Health Letter, December 30, 2017, http://www.health.harvard.edu/staying-healthy/blue-light-has-a-dark-side.

23 https://www.aarp.org/health/conditions-treatments/info-2016/sleep-apnea-insomnia.html

24 David Dudley, "World War ZZZ," *AARP Magazine*, August/September 2016, 55–58.

25 Cris Rowan, "10 Reasons Why Handheld Devices Should Be Banned for Children under the Age of 12," *Huffington Post*, March 6, 2014, http://www.huffingtonpost.com/cris-rowan/10-reasons-why-handheld-devices-should-be-banned_b_4899218.html.

26 Docket file copy original, Federal Communications Commission, 2016, https://ecfsapi.fcc.gov/file/60001421596.pdf.

27 *Generation Zapped*, official trailer from Sabine El Gemayel on Vimeo, https://player.vimeo.com/video/221492864?inf_contact_key=d174fdd07f0d4a4cbce3b8d0232a673acc42e391404745ac10e061328cb6b0a2.

28 Diane Ostermann, "Wireless or Not, Smart Meters Harm Your Health." Michigan Stop Smart Meters, November 2012, https://michiganstopsmartmeters.com/wireless-or-not-smart-meters-harm-your-health/.

29 J. R. Thorpe, "5 Things Too Much Screen Time Does to Your Body," Bustle, October 26, 2015, https://www.bustle.com/articles/117838-5-things-too-much-screen-time-does-to-your-body.

30 Twenge, *iGen: Why Today's Super Connected Kids Are Growing Up Less Rebellious, More Tolerant, Less Happy*, 176.

31 Council on Communications and Media, "Virtual Violence," *Pediatrics*, July 2016, http://pediatrics.aappublications.org/content/early/2016/07/14/peds.2016-1298.

32 Lindsey Tanner, "Rising Teen Suicides and a Surge in Social Media Use. Is There a Link?" *Time*, November 14, 2017, https://www.msn.com/en-us/health/wellness/rising-teen-suicides-and-a-surge-in-social-media-use-is-there-a-link/ar-BBEWBqI?ocid=sf.

33 Jean Twenge, Thomas Joiner, Megan Rogers, et al., "Increases in Depressive Symptoms, Suicide-Related Outcomes, and Suicide Rates Among U.S. Adolescents After 2010 and Links to Increased New Media Screen Time," *Clinical Psychological Science* 6 (2017): 3–17. doi: 10.1177/2167702617723376.

34 Twenge, *iGen Why Today's Super Connected Kids Are Growing Up Less Rebellious, More Tolerant, Less Happy*, 71, 72.

35 Tanner, "Rising Teen Suicides and a Surge in Social Media Use."

36 "Aw Shit, the Author of the Llama Llama Books Died of Cancer at Age 50," youbemom.com forum, September 7, 2016, https://www.youbemom.com/forum/permalink/8717726/aw-shit-the-author-of-the-llama-llama-books-died-of-cancer-at-age.

37 Healy, *Endangered Minds*, 102.

38 Perri Klass, "Bedtime Stories for Young Brains," *New York Times*, Well blog, August 17, 2015, http://well.blogs.nytimes.com/2015/08/17/bedtime-stories-for-young-brains/.

39 http://kodaheart.com/10-things-21/

40 Michele Borba, *UnSelfie: Why Empathetic Kids Succeed in Our All-about-Me World* (New York: Touchstone, 2017), 77.

41 Klass, "Bedtime Stories for Young Brains."

42 Michelle Borba, "UnSelfie," 2016, http://micheleborba.com/tag/unselfie/.

43 "Selected Research on Screen Time and Children," Campaign for a Commercial-Free Childhood.

44 Victoria Dunckley, "The Radical Notion of Returning to Handwriting," Psychology Today, May 2017, https://www.psychologytoday.com/blog/mental-wealth/201705/the-radical-notion-returning-handwriting.

45 Dunckley, "The Radical Notion of Returning to Handwriting."

46 Perri Klass, "Why Handwriting Is Still Essential in the Keyboard Age," *New York Times*, Well blog, June 20, 2016, https://well.blogs.nytimes.com/2016/06/20/why-handwriting-is-still-essential-in-the-keyboard-age/.

47 Twenge, *iGen Why Today's Super Connected Kids Are Growing Up Less Rebellious, More Tolerant, Less Happy*, 63, 64.

48 "Selected Research on Screen Time and Children," Campaign for a Commercial-Free Childhood.

49 Samantha Guzman, "How Screen Addiction Is Hurting Children," KERA News, August 17, 2016, http://keranews.org/post/how-screen-addiction-hurting-children.

50 Caitlin Emma, "Finland's Low-Tech Take on Education," POLITICO, May 27, 2014, http://www.politico.com/story/2014/05/finland-school-system-107137.

51 Jean Yung, "China's Challenges," *GlobalPost*, April 13, 2010, https://www.globalpost.com/dispatch/education/100407/technology-the-classroom-chinas-challenges.

52 Chris Weller, "Bill Gates and Steve Jobs Raised Their Kids Tech-Free—and It Should've been a Red Flag," *Business Insider*, January 10, 2018, www.businessinsider.com/screen-time-limits-bill-gates-steve-jobs-red-flag-2017-10.

53 Alex Hern, "'Never Get High on Your Own Supply'—Why Social Media Bosses Don't Use Social Media," *The Guardian*, January 23, 2018, https://www.theguardian.com/media/2018/jan/23/never-get-high-on-your-own-supply-why-social-media-bosses-dont-use-social-media.

54 Luke Kawa, "Two Major Apple Shareholders Push for Study of IPhone Addiction in Children," *Bloomberg*, January 7, 2018, https://www.bloomberg.com/news/articles/2018-01-08/jana-calpers-push-apple-to-study-iphone-addiction-in-children.

55 "CrazyBusy," Dr Hallowell, Live a Better Life, 2009, http://www.drhallowell.com/crazy-busy/.

56 Jennifer Hoffman, "Watch Out! Visual Concentration Can Leave You Temporarily 'Deaf'," ABC News, December 8, 2015, http://abcnews.go.com/Health/watch-visual-concentration-leave-temporarily-deaf/story?id=35650144.

57 Guzman, "How Screen Addiction Is Hurting Children."

58 Joshua Krisch, "Why Online Gamers Perform Better in School," Vocativ, August 8, 2016, http://www.vocativ.com/348731/why-online-gamers-perform-better-in-school/.

59 "Video Games Help Doctors Improve Surgical Skills," Florida Hospital press release, August 22, 2016, https://www.floridahospital.com/news/video-games-help-doctors-improve-surgical-skills.

60 "What Makes a Video Game Addictive?" Video Game Addiction, 2008, http://www.video-game-addiction.org/what-makes-games-addictive.html.

61 "Why Won't My Child Stop Playing Video Games?" Video Game Addiction, 2008, http://www.video-game-addiction.org/note2.html.

62 Cris Rowan, "Technology Myth and Fact Sheet," Moving to Learn, January 7, 2016, http://movingtolearn.ca/2016/technology-myth-and-fact-sheet.

63 Nicole Crawford, "Wired Kids: How Screen Time Affects Children's Brains," Breaking Muscle, 2013, http://breakingmuscle.com/family-kids/wired-kids-how-screen-time-affects-childrens-brains.

64 Kardaras, "It's 'Digital Heroin.'"

65 Kardaras, "It's 'Digital Heroin.'"

66 "Video Game Addiction Is Real. BEWARE!" Andrew Doan, Facebook, 2015, https://www.facebook.com/DrAndrewDoan/videos/838608992864375/.

67 Kardaras, "It's 'Digital Heroin.'"

68 Conor Duffy, "Screen Addiction: Health Experts Say Excessive Amounts of Time Spent on Phones, Tablets Can Affect Childhood Development," ABC News (Australia), January 27, 2014, http://www.abc.net.au/news/2014-01-27/screen-addiction-experts-raise-concerns/5221278.

69 "What Makes a Video Game Addictive?" Video Game Addiction.

70 Twenge, *iGen Why Today's Super Connected Kids Are Growing Up Less Rebellious, More Tolerant, Less Happy*, 51.

71 Cris Rowan, "When Parents Prefer Devices," Moving to Learn, November 6, 2015, http://movingtolearn.ca/2015/when-parents-prefer-devices.

72 Laurel Wamsley, "France Moves to Ban Students from Using Cellphones in Schools," NPR, December 12, 2017, https://www.npr.org/sections/thetwo-way/2017/12/12/570145408/france-moves-to-ban-students-from-using-cellphones-in-schools.

73 Rachel Macy Stafford, "Tether Yourself: The Enlightening Talk Parents Aren't Having Can Keep Teens from a Damaging Drift," Hands Free Mama blog, December 12, 2015, https://www.handsfreemama.com/2017/12/15/tether-yourself-the-enlightening-talk-parents-arent-having-can-keep-teens-from-a-damaging-drift/.

74 "Media and Children," American Academy of Pediatrics, September 9, 2016, https://www.aap.org/en-us/advocacy-and-policy/aap-health-initiatives/Pages/Media-and-Children.aspx?rf=32524.

75 Rowan, "10 Reasons Why Handheld Devices Should Be Banned for Children Under the Age of 12."

76 Melissa Kirsch, "Change Your Screen to Grayscale to Combat Phone Addiction," Lifehacker.com, June 5, 2017, https://lifehacker.com/change-your-screen-to-grayscale-to-combat-phone-addicti-1795821843.

77 Victoria Dunckley, *Reset Your Child's Brain: A Four-Week Plan to End Meltdowns, Raise Grades, and Boost Social Skills by Reversing the Effects of Electronic Screen-Time* (Novato, CA: New World Library, 2015).

Chapter seven

1 Kathryn Vasel, "Working from Home Is Really Having a Moment," CNN Money, June 21, 2017, money.cnn.com/2017/06/21/pf/jobs/working-from-home/index.html.

2 Elizabeth McGrory, "4 Reasons Why Companies Need to Be More Flexible with Working Parents," The Spruce, February 2017, https://www.thespruce.com/reasons-why-companies-need-to-be-more-flexible-4125217.

3 "How Many Times Does the Average American Move?" Reference.com, September 3, 2016, https://www.reference.com/health/many-times-average-american-move-e8e3a9c6af3327f5.

4   Daniel Moore, "Should Workers Be Compensated for Answering Emails, Texts, Calls on Mobile When Off-the-Clock?" *Pittsburgh Post-Gazette*, October 15, 2015, www.post-gazette.com/business/career-workplace/2015/10/18/Should-workers-be-compensated-for-answering-emails-texts-calls-on-mobile-when-off-the-clock/stories/201510180049.

5   Edward Hallowell, *CrazyBusy: Overstretched, Overbooked, and About to Snap!* (New York: Ballantine Books, 2006), 57.

6   Katie Hurley, "4 Reasons to Stop Rushing Your Kids," EverydayFamily, January 2014, https://www.everydayfamily.com/blog/4-reasons-to-stop-rushing-your-kids/#.

7   "The Film, The Movement." *Race to Nowhere*, www.racetonowhere.com/about-film.

8   Gary Small, "Is Technology Fracturing Your Family?" Psychology Today, June 19, 2009, https://www.psychologytoday.com/blog/brain-bootcamp/200906/is-technology-fracturing-your-family.

9   "Why Kids Need Routines," Aha! Parenting, www.ahaparenting.com/parenting-tools/family-life/structure-routines.

10   Matt Richtel, "The Competing Views on Competition," *New York Times*, October 10, 2012, https://www.nytimes.com/2012/10/11/garden/the-role-of-competitiveness-in-raising-healthy-children.html.

11   "6 Benefits of Family Time," Family Focus blog, 2013, http://familyfocusblog.com/6-benefits-of-spending-time-together-as-a-family/.

Chapter eight

1   "Why Parenting Styles Matter When Raising Children by Kendra Cherry," book review by Steven Gans, Verywell, https://www.verywell.com/parenting-styles-2795072.

2   Bianca Mgbemere and Rachel Telles, "Types of Parenting Styles and How to Identify Yours," Developmental Psychology at Vanderbilt, https://my.vanderbilt.edu/developmentalpsychologyblog/2013/12/types-of-parenting-styles-and-how-to-identify-yours/.

3   Gwen Dewar, "Parenting Styles: A Guide for the Science-Minded," Parenting Science—The Science of Child-Rearing and Child Development, https://www.parentingscience.com/parenting-styles.html.

4   Brendan Smith, "The Case against Spanking," Monitor on Psychology, American Psychological Association, www.apa.org/monitor/2012/04/spanking.aspx/.

5   "4 Parenting Styles—Characteristics and Effects," Parenting for Brain, October 8, 2017, https://www.parentingforbrain.com/4-baumrind-parenting-styles/.

6   David Hosier, "Childhood Trauma: The Possible Effects of Uninvolved Parents," Childhood Trauma Recovery, January 17, 2014, https://childhoodtraumarecovery.com/2014/01/17/childhood-trauma-the-possible-effects-of-uninvolved-parents/.

7   Michele Borba, "Seven Deadly Parenting Styles," Dr. Michele Borba, June 13, 2012, micheleborba.com/7-deadly-parenting-styles-of-modern-day-child-rearing/.

8   Michelle Borba, *UnSelfie: Why Empathetic Kids Succeed in Our All-About-Me World* (New York: Touchstone, 2016), jacket cover.

9   Borba. *UnSelfie*, xii.

10   Borba, *UnSelfie*, 195.

11   "Resilience," Merriam-Webster, https://www.merriam-webster.com/dictionary/resilience.

12   "Grit," Merriam-Webster, https://www.merriam-webster.com/dictionary/grit.

13   "Building Resilience in Children and Teens," Fostering Resilience, fosteringresilience.com/books.php.

14   "Dr. Kenneth R. Ginsburg's 7 Crucial C's of Resilience," SchoolQuest, 2013, https://www.schoolquest.org/blog/entry/dr.-kenneth-r.-ginsburgs-7crucial-cs-of-resilience.

15   Mary Beth Hicks, *Bringing Up Geeks: Genuine, Enthusiastic, Empowered Kids* (New York: Penguin Books, 2008), 200–201.

16   "Olweus Bullying Prevention Program," Violence Prevention Works, 2012, https://www.violencepreventionworks.org/public/olweus_bullying_prevention_program.page.

17   Wendy Mogul, *The Blessing of a Skinned Knee: Using Jewish Teachings to Raise Self-Reliant Children* (New York: Scribner, 2008).

Chapter nine

1   "Children and Sleep," National Sleep Foundation, sleepfoundation.org/sleep-topics/children-and-sleep.

2   Eric Olson, "How Many Hours of Sleep Do You Need?" Mayo Clinic, April 6, 2016, https://www.mayoclinic.org/healthy-lifestyle/adult-health/expert-answers/how-many-hours-of-sleep-are-enough/faq-20057898.

3   Chris Rowan, "Sustainable Children: Are They a Blast from the Past?" Moving to Learn, June 17, 2016, http://movingtolearn.ca/2016/sustainable-children-are-they-a-blast-from-the-past.

4   Megan Waltz, "The Importance of Social and Emotional Development in Young Children," Ready 4 K, January 2013, http://childrensacademyonline.net/wp-content/uploads/2013/01/Importance-of-SEL-In-Early-Childhood-Devt.pdf.

5   Karen Dickinson and Rick Parsons, *A Student's Guide to Stress Management* (San Diego: Cognella, 2018).

6   "The Causes & Symptoms of Stress," The Cortisol Connection, cortisol.com/causes-symptoms-stress/#.Wn5KGJPwYdU.

7   Linda Gabriel, "BDNF—Miracle-Gro for the Brain," Thought Medicine, May 2010, thoughtmedicine.com/2010/05/bdnf-miracle-gro-for-the-brain/.

8   "Average Attention Span by Age," Day 2 Day Parenting, October 21, 2015, day2dayparenting.com/qa-normal-attention-span/.

9   Perri Klass, "Bedtime Stories for Young Brains," *New York Times*, Well blog, August 17, 2015, http://well.blogs.nytimes.com/2015/08/17/bedtime-stories-for-young-brains/.

10   Mary Anne Duggan and Larissa Gaias, "Raising Arizona Kids," *Raising Arizona Kids Magazine*, April 2013, https://www.raisingarizonakids.com/2013/04/the-fourth-r-of-early-school-success-self-regulation/.

11   "An Introduction to 'How Does Your Engine Run?'" The Alert Program, https://www.alertprogram.com/?s=how+does+your+engine+run?.

12   Kathy Hirsch-Pasek and Roberta Michnick Golinkoff, *Einstein Never Used Flashcards: How Our Children Really Learn—and Why They Need to Play More and Memorize Less* (Emmaus, PA: Rodale, 2003).

13   Joshua Becker, "Why Fewer Toys Will Benefit Your Kids," Becoming Minimalist blog, 2011, http://www.becomingminimalist.com/why-fewer-toys-will-actually-benefit-your-kids/.

14   John J. Ratey, "Run, Jump, Learn! How Exercise can Transform Our Schools," TEDx, November 18, 2012, https://www.youtube.com/watch?v=hBSVZdTQmDs.

15   Shelley Frost, "Why Is It Important to Develop Gross Motor Skills in Preschool Children?" Livestrong, June 13, 2017, https://www.livestrong.com/article/179169-why-is-it-important-to-develop-gross-motor-skills-in-preschool-children/.

16   "Heavy Work Activities (Proprioceptive Input) ... They Need Them, They Crave Them!" Heavy Work Activities, https://www.sensory-processing-disorder.com/heavy-work-activities.html.

17   "40 Heavy Work Activities for Kids," Mama OT, April 7, 2015, http://mamaot.com/40-heavy-work-activities-kids/.

18   "Develop Your Child's Brain with Swimming," Swim Kids USA, December 19, 2012, www.swimkidsaz.com/blog/develop-your-childs-brain-with-swimming/.

19   Susan Thompson, *Handy Learning: Activities for Hand Development and Curriculum Enhancement* (Flower Mound, TX: Handy Learning Seminars, Inc., 2008), 7.

20   Anna Ranson, "40 Fine Motor Skills Activities," The Imagination Tree, September 3, 2013, https://theimaginationtree.com/40-fine-motor-skills-activities-for-kids/.

21   Amanda Hermes, "Sand & Water Play for Infants & Toddlers," Livestrong, June 13, 2017, https://www.livestrong.com/article/287562-sand-water-play-for-infants-toddlers/.

22   Michele Borba, *UnSelfie: Why Empathetic Kids Succeed in Our All-about-Me World* (New York: Touchstone, 2017), 7.

23   Borba, *UnSelfie*, 183, 184.

24 Sally Deneen, "Mind–Body Connection," SUCCESS, April 4, 2010, https://www.success.com/article/mind-body-connection.

25 Maria Popova, "How Playing Music Benefits Your Brain More than Any Other Activity," Brain Pickings, January 29, 2015, https://www.brainpickings.org/2015/01/29/music-brain-ted-ed/.

26 Naomi Coleman, "Three More Health Benefits of Being beside the Sea," Daily Mail Online, November 15, 2002, http://www.dailymail.co.uk/health/article-102698/Three-health-benefits-sea.html.

27 Cris Rowan, "Unplug—Don't Drug: A Critical Look at the Influence of Technology on Child Behavior with an Alternative Way of Responding Other than Evaluation and Drugging," Constant Contact, July 2016, http://archive.constantcontact.com/fs193/1101930228564/archive/1124533850807.html.

28 "150 Conversation Starters for Family Discussions," Aha! Parenting, 2009, http://www.ahaparenting.com/parenting-tools/communication/family-discussions.

29 Jenny Williams, "What Is Grit, Why Kids Need It, and How You Can Foster It," A Fine Parent, 2015, https://afineparent.com/building-character/what-is-grit.html.

30 Carol Dweck, "Carol Dweck Revisits the 'Growth Mindset,'" Education Week, September 23, 2015, https://www.edweek.org/ew/articles/2015/09/23/carol-dweck-revisits-the-growth-mindset.html.

31 Amanda Morin, "Why Cognitive Skill Milestones Are Important for Your Child," Verywell Family, December 26, 2017, https://www.verywellfamily.com/what-are-cognitive-skills-620847.

32 Morin, "Why Cognitive Skill Milestones Are Important for Your Child."

33 Willy Wood (Columbia, MO)—Weebly, blog, September 19, 2017.

34 Ana Prana, "Superbrain Yoga: 3 Minutes That Maximize Brain Power," Collective Evolution, September 6, 2015, https://www.collective-evolution.com/2015/09/06/superbrain-yoga-3-minutes-that-maximize-brain-power/.

35 Dr. Ramesh, "Super Brain Yoga: A Research Study," 2013, http://guruprasad.net/wp-content/uploads/2013/12/sby-a-research-study.pdf.

36 "The Health Benefits of Strong Relationships," Harvard Women's Health Watch, December 2010, https://www.health.harvard.edu/newsletter_article/the-health-benefits-of-strong-relationships.

37 M. V. Fields and D. M. Fields, "How Children Develop Social Competence," Education.com, October 25, 2010, https://www.education.com/reference/article/children-develop-social-competence/.

38 "Understanding the Distracted," National Safety Council, 2014, http://www.nsc.org/DistractedDrivingDocuments/Cognitive-Distraction-White-Paper.pdf.

39 "Texting and Driving Statistics," TextingandDrivingSafety.com, 2012, http://www.textinganddrivingsafety.com/texting-and-driving-stats.

40 "Risk & Protective Factors," Youth.gov, https://youth.gov/youth-topics/substance-abuse/risk-and-protective-factors-substance-use-abuse-and-dependence.

41 Jean Twenge, *iGen: Why Today's Super-Connected Kids Are Growing up Less Rebellious, More Tolerant, Less Happy—and Completely Unprepared for Adulthood (and What This Means for the Rest of Us)* (New York: Atria Books, 2017).

42 Deneen, "Mind–Body Connection."

43 "Mirror Neurons and Athletes: Learning by Watching," Axon Sports, 2011, http://www.axonpotential.com/mirror-neurons-and-athletes/.

Chapter ten

1 "What Is Sensory Integration," Sense Able Kids, http://senseablekids.com/sensInt.html.

2 "Sensory Integration Dysfunction Symptoms: What You Must Know!" Sensory Processing Disorder (SPD), https://www.sensory-processing-disorder.com/sensory-integration-dysfunction-symptoms.html.

3 "Forbrain—Auditory Feedback Headset for Speech, Language and Attention," https://www.forbrain.com.

4 "The TOMATIS® Method." Tomatis® Method, Auditory Stimulation Program for Improving Brain Functions, https://www.tomatis.com/en.

5 Scientific Learning, https://www.scilearn.com.

6 "Welcome to the Able Kids Foundation," Able Kids Foundation, https://www.ablekidsfoundation.org.

7 "Lindamood-Bell Instruction," Lindamood-Bell, https://lindamoodbell.com/instruction.

8 "Study Cites Gray Matter Volume Changes Following Lindamood-Bell Instruction," Education Update Online, September/October 2011, educationupdate.com/archives/2011/SEP/HTML/spec-study.html.

9 Julie Gunter, "How the UW Helped a Little Girl Triumph as a Reader with Dyslexia," *Columns Magazine*, September 28, 2017, https://magazine.washington.edu/feature/dyslexia/.

10 "UW Study Examines How the Brains of Students with Dyslexia Respond to Intensive Reading Intervention (Seeing Stars)," Lindamood-Bell, October 13, 2017, https://lindamoodbell.com/research/uw-study-examines-brains-students-dyslexia-respond-intensive-reading-intervention-seeing-stars.

11 D. Corydon Hammond, "What Is Neurofeedback: An Update," *Journal of Neurotherapy* 15 (2011), www.isnr-jnt.org/article/view/16553/10521.

12 Interactive Metronome, https://www.interactivemetronome.com.

13 "A Mind-Body Stress-Reduction Technique," NET Mind Body, www.net-mindbody.com.

14 EMDR Institute, www.emdr.com.

15 "About," Jesse Lewis Choose Love Movement, https://www.jesselewischooselove.org/about-us/.

16 The Tapping Practice, https://www.thetappingpractice.com.

17 Integrative Medicine Academy, https://integrativemedicineacademy.com.

18 "What Is Integrative Medicine?" Arizona Center for Integrative Medicine, https://integrativemedicine.arizona.edu/about/definition.html.

19 Danielle Graham, "Genetics, Epigenetics, and Destiny: Interview with Dr. Bruce Lipton," *SuperConsciousness Magazine*, March 16, 2010, www.superconsciousness.com/topics/science/interview-dr-bruce-lipton.

20 "The Methylation Cycle." Dr. Amy Yasko, www.dramyyasko.com/our-unique-approach/methylation-cycle/.

21 "Acupuncture," Mayo Clinic, February 14, 2018, https://www.mayoclinic.org/tests-procedures/acupuncture/basics/definition/PRC-20020778.

22 "Massage These Stress Points to Immediately Relax a Fussy or Crying Baby," Shareably, https://shareably.co/foot-reflexology/.

Conclusion

1   "An Ambulance Down in the Valley," Independent Living, Inc., 2014, http://www.myindependentliving.org/NA-NewsArticles/AnAmbulanceDownInTheValley.

2   "Kathy Hirsh-Pasek," Play and Playground Encyclopedia, https://www.pgpedia.com/h/kathy-hirsh-pasek.

3   Documenting Hope, https://documentinghope.com.

Acknowledgments

We would like to thank Allyson Machate and Carl Lennertz who helped us in the early stages of this journey and the team at Cognella for the support and dedication needed to bring this book to fruition! We have been blessed with friends, family, and colleagues who have also contributed their wealth of experiences and expertise to make this book a valuable resource. We know that without their contributions and support, this book would not have been possible, and we hope that they will be happy with the final product. To all of you, please accept our appreciation and gratitude for your help and support:

Denise Currier, OD, practitioner of pediatric visual evaluations and therapy

Holly Grimm, LCSW, and Todd Grimm, LPC, board certified practitioners in neurofeedback

Christine Hannafin, PhD, NCC, LPC, and certified NET practitioner

Chaya Herzberg, OD, FCOVD, practitioner of pediatric visual evaluations and therapy

Lindsay LaRiviere, MEd, Lindamood Bell Center Executive Director

Maude LeRoux, OTR/L, SIPT, RCTC, DIR® Expert Trainer, A Total Approach

Lori Leyden, PhD, MBA, founder of Create Global Healing, trauma healing expert, transformational leader, and author

Moira Mahr, MEd, Pacific Grove Unified School District, Pacific Grove, CA

Janet McGaurn, DC, practitioner of chiropractic care

Oscar J. Martinez, MD

Nathalie Matte, DC, NRT practitioner

Jean Blaydes Moize, MEd, honorary PhD in Education, founder of Action Based Learning

Peter Prociuk, MD, practitioner of homeopathy

Suzanne Rossini, MEd, certified EFT practitioner

About the Authors

Monica Reinhard-Gorney, M.S.Ed. is a wife, mother of two girls, and a proprietor of a private educational counseling practice. Her counseling encompasses helping local students, as well as those around the globe, prepare for undergraduate and graduate school visits, interviews, and the overall higher education application process. Monica also helps to connect students and parents with educational resources and interventions to increase school success in grades K-12. She has worked in top private and public schools and holds a master's degree in school counseling from the University of Pennsylvania.

Perk Musacchio, M.Ed. is a wife, a mother of three, grandmother of four, and the owner of Skills2Soar, LLC, an educational consulting company. She has over 40 years of experience working with students of varying cognitive abilities, emotional needs, learning styles and disabilities, mastery of the English language, and levels of autism. Working with diverse populations has provided Perk with extensive experience in the areas of curriculum and program development, instructional techniques, behavior management strategies, crisis prevention and intervention, leadership, and professional development and consultation. She earned her master's degree in education from Temple University.

34335954R10183

Made in the USA
Columbia, SC
15 November 2018